Natural pregnancy

A green guide to the
most important nine months
of your life

Susannah Marriott

CARROLL & BROWN PUBLISHERS LIMITED

First published in 2006 in the United Kingdom by

Carroll & Brown Publishers Limited
20 Lonsdale Road London NW6 6RD

Design Simon Daley, Emily Cook & Laura de Grasse

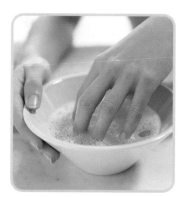

Text © Susannah Marriott 2005
Illustrations and compilation © Carroll & Brown Limited 2005

A CIP catalogue record for this book is available from the
British Library.

ISBN 1-904760-45-7
ISBN-13 978-1-904760-45-0

10987654321

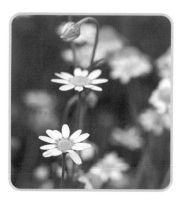

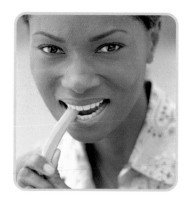

Reproduced by RALI, Bilbao, Spain
Printed and bound by Bookprint, S.L., Barcelona

Contents

Introduction

We are surrounded by manmade chemicals. The computer in front of me is pumping out contaminated dust, so reports say; the water I'm sipping is chlorinated; the banana and coffee I'm enjoying may be laced with pesticide residues; and I daren't consider the gunk I slathered over my hair, body and face when getting dressed this morning. Toothpaste, clothing, mattresses and sofas, indoor air – all could contain traces of noxious substances.

Should we be concerned, especially during pregnancy when there's so much other stuff to fret about – alcohol, cigarettes, soft cheese? Why would we want to worry about the cleaners and air fresheners that ensure an instant sparkling bath or forest-fresh living room when we're so lacking in energy but so big on nesting?

Everyone alive – and all newborn babies tested – has measurable levels of synthetic chemicals in the body. It's been estimated that every American has, on average, a store of 100 industrial and agricultural chemicals. Many build up in body fat faster than our detox systems can get rid of them. Many pass through the placenta to the baby. Some scramble the hormones that trigger normal development. If we wait to start worrying until it's time to choose organic food at weaning, we could be missing the boat.

We can't escape these substances since they infect every part of our environment – the soil our food is grown in, our water supplies, our most remote areas. Even those banned decades ago persist because they don't break down easily.

But don't despair or stop reading. There is plenty you can do. This book provides dozens of recipes for homemade products of all types that are free of dangerous toxins. It also counsels on what to eat, and to create a home environment that is safe and supportive. Throughout the book, you'll find recommendations for innovative products that are safe during pregnancy made by the good guys (actually, often caring mums). Some are from the UK, many from the US, others Dutch or Kiwi – a network of alternative living stretches across the globe and, thanks to the Web, it's easy to hook up and join in, wherever you live.

The book also suggests ways to build up your body and mind better to withstand the aches, pains and worries that only add to the stress (because that's toxic, too), such as yoga, massage and meditation. The most important thing is to enjoy your pregnancy, because the less stress you suffer the less risk to your baby. So go get that fabulous organic chocolate and untreated silk maternity wear. Get your purse out, because the fight for your money is where all this begins and ends. By buying good products – like organic food and paints that aren't made from dodgy ingredients – and avoiding nasty products you get to change the world for the better. Just a little bit, but day by day, life by life, and home by home, this ameliorates the way we all live. As shoppers we have the power to demand change – look how British consumers deterred supermarkets from stocking GM foods.

Who am I to advocate this? I'm the alarmed mother of three young daughters trying to bring to a wider audience guidance on what is safe and what is not during pregnancy. I did plenty of research during my own pregnancies: the first one switched

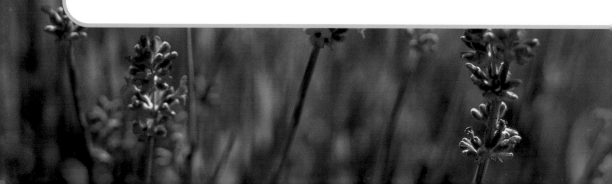

me on to organic food; the second, eco cosmetics; third time around it was the mattress thing. After writing this, I'm moving out of London to live by the sea in Cornwall!

Some of the information here is controversial; most of it isn't mentioned in conventional pregnancy manuals. This doesn't mean you might not (should not) be interested. Enough experts are worrying about the health implications for you and your baby of our toxic world. And isn't this the time in life when you want to be most protected and most protective? Whether the science around the health risks is well-defined or not.

Who else cares? Aware celebs, like Sarah Jessica Parker and Gwyneth Paltrow, who won't give up the glamour to be clean and green, and so shop during pregnancy at organic cosmetic emporia such as London's Organic Pharmacy. And the UK's leading scientific agency, the Royal Society, who in 2000, urged "it is prudent to minimize exposure of humans [to hormone-disrupting pesticides], especially pregnant women".

So be concerned, but don't be scared. In the end, there's a positive message: you can make a difference to your own good health – and that of your own precious baby.

Susannah Marriott

Protecting the next generation

Throwing up your hands in horror? Here are the best ways to start making a difference.

* Eat organic food.
* Fit a water filter.
* Stop anyone smoking in your home.
* Detox your bathroom cabinet and makeup bag: especially get rid of aerosols.
* Buy green cleaning and laundry products.
* Take off your shoes at the door so you don't tread in pesticides.
* Clear out chemicals in your garden shed.
* Don't use clingfilm or buy plastic-packed readymeals.
* Chuck out air "fresheners". Open windows to air your home instead.
* Investigate organic sheets and clothing, mattresses and paint.
* Stop toxic thoughts (and widen your pelvis) with pregnancy yoga.

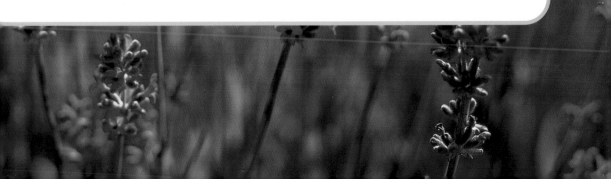

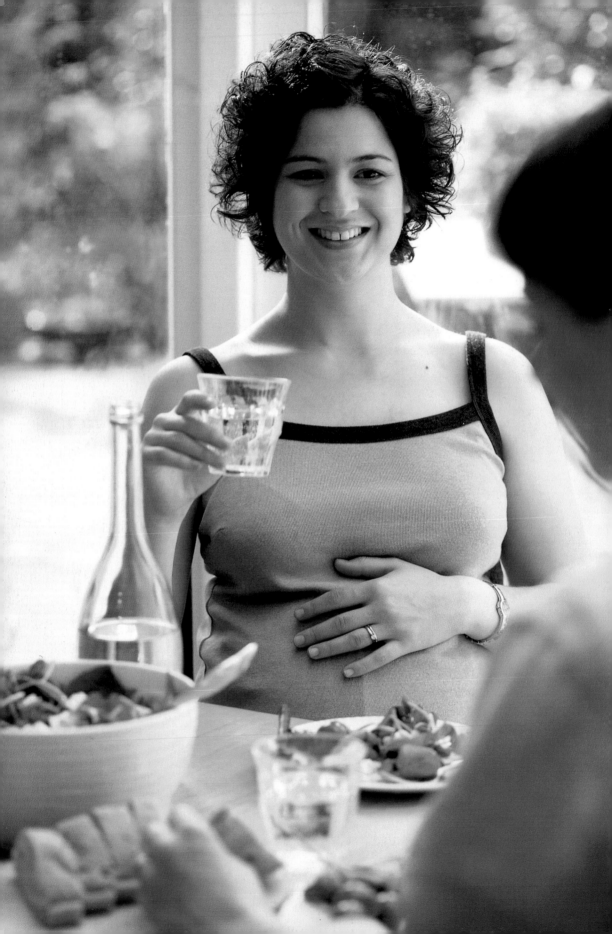

Pure food

A human baby is the supreme example of you are what you eat! The right food at the right time safeguards your baby's healthy development not only in the womb but as he grows into adulthood, helping reduce the risk of asthma, heart disease and certain forms of cancer. A good diet is good for you, too, easing common pregnancy ailments, from nausea to heartburn, and reducing the risk of pregnancy complications – even premature birth. But your baby is also vulnerable to the negative effects of toxins in food. This chapter explains how to shield yourself and your baby with a diet that contains all the essential nutrients that can ensure your pregnancy is as healthy as it can possibly be.

Eating to protect your baby

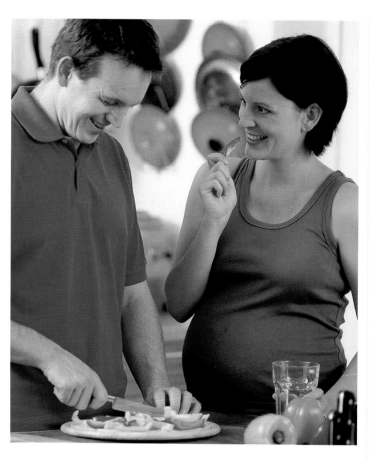

Choose organic

Certified organic food means not only a lower risk of dining on pesticide residues (organic farmers manage the land with minimal agrochemicals), crops and livestock raised organically are more likely to have been looked after by people who value the health of the soil, encourage biodiversity, restore indigenous habitats to benefit wildlife and cause less pollution to water sources, making the environment healthier for everyone, including your baby. Doesn't that makes every mouthful more palatable? Choosing fairtraded organic goods, such as cocoa and bananas, ensures workers in developing countries don't have to be exposed to toxic chemicals and that their children's healthcare needs are provided for, too. The UK's Soil Association permits only 29 additives to be added to processed organic foods, such as sausages and ice cream: some 500 are sanctioned for use in conventional products. Organic foods also are certified free from GM material. Genetic modification seeks to change substances at a molecular level, copying genes from one plant or animal to another. As well as the obvious ethical questions this poses, there may be health implications for our flora and fauna as well as for those who eat the resulting food.

Fresh organic food can be flavour-intensive and some studies have shown it to be higher in

Feeding your baby doesn't start with breastfeeding; it begins before conception. What you eat builds your baby's body, so make sure it's the best you can find: sensitivity to potentially damaging chemicals is much higher while your child is in the womb and newborn than at any time in childhood. The first priority for low-tox living is to buy and eat food in as natural a state as possible – choose a fresh organic apple over canned pineapple, top-quality streak over processed pies, homebaked rather than takeaway. Changing your diet is one of the best, easiest and most enjoyable ways to reduce your risk of low-level exposure to toxins known to have adverse effects on reproductive health and the development of unborn babies. Even if eating organic doesn't reduce your current body stores of toxins, it reduces toxins in the environment. For these few months, don't compromise on quality and you might even find you suffer less sleepless nights, too.

minerals and vitamins C, A and E. The extra staffing and care needed to produce it also make it more expensive.

You don't have to convert to a totally organic diet at once. Try adding a few staples to your shopping basket each week. And when given the option of organic food from the other side of the world versus a non-organic product from your local farmer's market, go local, questioning the seller (often the farmer) about his farming methods.

Where should I shop?

Think beyond the organic aisle of your regular supermarket. A small producer is more likely to care about the quality of the food from (his) fork to (your) fork, and the

best way to meet him or her is by shopping at farm stores or farmer's markets (where 40-60 percent of producers are likely to be organic, according to US research). Ask how livestock is raised, cheeses made and fruit grown. Try also specialist organic supermarkets and health food stores.

Support local greengrocers, fishmongers and butchers, quizzing them about their sources and encouraging them to stock the items you want.

Find out about organic box schemes – some companies deliver everything from juices to meat. Also good are Web-based delivery services direct from the farm gate or quay.

In the UK, if you can't afford organic everything, shop for the rest at Marks and Spencer or Co-

Psst... Passing the placenta Certain common pesticides – organophosphates – travel readily across the placenta into the unborn baby as was proved by laboratory studies at Bristol University. But researchers at the University of Washington found that children who ate organic food had significantly lower levels of the breakdown products of OP pesticides in their bodies. Eating organic, therefore, exposes your baby to less risk.

op, supermarkets that have acted to ban controversial pesticides. (Waitrose makes good efforts, too).

Eat seasonal, eat fresh

Good ingredients need least preparation, making for healthy food fast: it is satisfyingly quick to assemble a spread of farmhouse cheeses, ripe tomatoes, crunchy salad leaves and crusty bread. The best-tasting produce is what's in season where you live right now. Seasonal ingredients picked and eaten fresh and ripe contain more vital nutrients and flavour-enhancing compounds.

Source your food locally to ensure maximum freshness and a smaller chance of it having been sprayed with post-harvest pesticides and waxes for safe travelling. Such food will have travelled fewer food

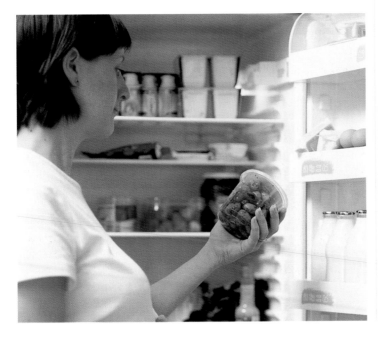

miles than most items in your supermarket, reducing the environmental pollution that might be harming your health as you breathe. Favour shops that mark the food miles on each product. Once you've found out what's local to you, have fun sampling it – wild game in season, regional apples and nuts, local raspberries and asparagus, speciality hard cheeses, artisan breads and glorious cakes and pastries.

What you need

Complex carbs

Forget low-carb regimes. For slow-release of energy to keep you on top of things and stave off nausea make bread, pasta, rice, oats, potatoes and pulses one third of your daily diet (4-6 portions a day) especially during the first trimester and when carbo-loading for birth in the last 6 weeks (like an athlete preparing to run a marathon). The fibre content helps the body process waste efficiently, helping prevent constipation and haemorrhoids.

Low-tox sources

Opt for whole unrefined organic grains that supply the B vitamins, iron and fibre stripped out of refined grains. In 2003, pesticide traces were found in 61 percent of UK bread sampled. A 1993 US study showed organically grown wheat had double the calcium, four times the magnesium and 13 times more selenium than conventional wheat. Choose organic bread from artisan bakers for best taste and to be sure it's free of artificial flour- or dough-improvers and bleaching agents. When buying non-organic bread, think French housewife; only buy fresh-baked loaves that go off after a day.

Fruit and vegetables

Source of vital vitamins, minerals and plant substances (phytochemicals) that have profound health benefits. Make these, too, a third of your diet by eating more than 5 portions a day.

Low-tox sources

Fruit If you need to make a choice, prioritize buying organic fruit – US studies show pesticide residues on fruit are higher than for any other type of produce. In 2003, all soft citrus fruit tested in the UK had residues – 96 percent from multiple sources. A University of California study found organic fruit contained 58 percent more antioxidants than conventionally grown produce. Organic fruit is not waxed with petrochemicals like most hard fruit, nor coated with postharvest fungicides to preserve lifespan.

Vegetables In UK tests, a quarter of spinach and more than a third of potatoes contained chemical residues. Organic spinach and cabbage, potatoes and lettuce not only avoid this risk, they have been shown to contain higher levels of minerals than their conventionally grown counterparts. Organic spinach, for example, has 100 percent more iron and manganese.

Simple ways to healthy foods

* Buy organic when you can, especially dairy foods and meat.
* Buy ethically to reduce pesticide use worldwide.
* Choose food sourced locally: it's likely to be fresher and more seasonal and will help reduce environmental toxins caused by planes, lorries and refrigeration.
* Scrub non-organic fruit and vegetables thoroughly with a nail brush specially reserved for this purpose and a squirt of green washing-up liquid. Rinse very well.
* Peel non-organic fruit and vegetables and remove outer leaves (though be aware that some pesticides penetrate the whole plant).
* Eat a wide variety of produce to reduce the risk of being exposed to the same pesticides many times.
* Email your supermarket asking about its policy on pesticide reduction and hormone-disrupting chemicals.

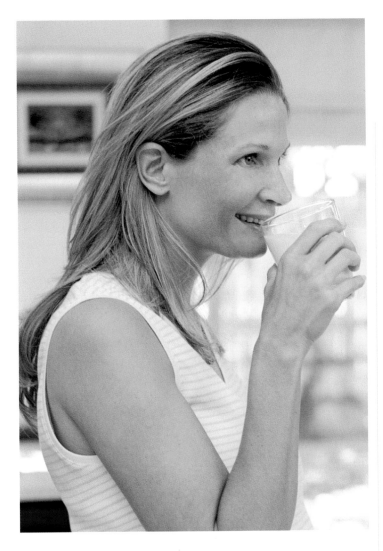

Organic carrots and potatoes don't need to be peeled – great because many of the goodies are in the skin. When you buy organic sweetcorn, you know it's not genetically modified, a worry when choosing US produce, and glossy vegetables won't be waxed.

Salad crops Choose organic prepacked salads, which are not chlorine-rinsed like their conventional counterparts; this can destroy vitamin content. Non-organic prepacked salad leaves contained the highest pesticide residues of all UK foods tested. Organic tomatoes and lettuce are grown in soil, rather than hydroponically and so may have a more homegrown texture and taste.

Dairy foods

Calcium, protein and B vitamins – make these a must during pregnancy. Milk, yogurt and cheese should be about 15 percent of your food intake (2-4 portions a day).

Low-tox choices

Since toxins accumulate in fat, organic dairy produce is your best choice – indeed, some dairy-intolerant women find they don't react to organic produce. Try semi-skimmed if you can't find organic: it has almost as much calcium as full-fat. Seek out old-fashioned glass milk bottles and a delivery man. Many natural health advocates recommend butter over margarine with its long lists of additives. Organically reared animals and those from small family farms are more likely to have been raised on pasture and dried feed rather than processed feed, and consequently their milk may retain more health-giving omega-3 fatty acids. A 2005 UK study found organic milk also had more vitamins A and E and was 75 percent higher in antioxidants than conventional milk. In the US, switch to organic or "No rBGH" milk and cheese, or select European brands to avoid hormone treatment. All pregnant women should avoid soft, unpasteurized and mould-ripened or blue-veined cheeses, which may be contaminated with the organism *Listeria monocytegenes*. In a tiny amount of cases, it can cause miscarriage and stillbirth. You might like also to avoid feta cheese. In 1999, 67 percent tested in the UK contained traces of DDT, a banned highly toxic hormone-disrupter.

Protein

As this provides the raw materials for a baby, you need much more than before pregnancy – about 12 percent of your daily food intake or 3-4 portions of meat, poultry, fish, nuts or pulses with whole grains a day. Its amino acids are the building blocks of every cell and tissue, and so the baby's muscles, organs, bones and hair. Protein sources also provide essential vitamins and minerals and keep your fluids well balanced.

Oily fish is an excellent source of omega-3 fatty acids, essential for a baby's brain and eye development, and eating fish appears to boost birthweight suggests a 2004 study by Bristol University (and so protect health in later life). Fish oils may even counteract the effects of air pollution on the heart. British women are urged to eat two portions of fish a week, one of them an oily fish.

Low-tox sources

If you can't source expensive wild salmon (which has 16 times less PCB [polychlorinated biphenyl] contamination than farmed salmon said a 2003 US report), choose organically farmed salmon and trout kept in waters monitored for purity and not fed artificial colourants, growth promoters or unnecessary antibiotics.

In North America, favour Canadian-caught fish and fish products: Canada rejects fish with half the level of methyl mercury allowed in US catches. For ocean fish, opt for rod and line-caught varieties from relatively unpolluted waters including off New Zealand and Argentina.

Self-caught American freshwater fish aren't recommended for pregnant women because of concerns about contamination in lakes and rivers.

To reduce your intake of mercury, PCBs, dioxins and other pollutants, observe the guidelines below and eat a variety of fish to spread the mix of contaminants. Unfortunately, in the end, it's left to you to weigh up the benefits of possible contamination with getting the nutrients you need.

Fish to consume any time (not overfished, farmed destructively or high in pollutants): Anchovies, herring, hoki, wild salmon, some organically farmed salmon, trout and catfish, sardines, Pacific squid, farmed bass and sturgeon.

Fish to consume less than once a month: Pollak, canned tuna, Pacific cod, Alaskan halibut, grouper, amberjack, mahi mahi and fatty fish products, such as caviar.

Fish to avoid: Carnivorous fish high on the foodchain, such as swordfish, shark, marlin, bluefin and albacore tuna, king mackerel, tilefish (golden bass or golden snapper), Atlantic halibut, pike; also avoid tuna steaks.

Don't eat raw fish, including sushi, sashimi, nor seared steaks.

Eggs Buy free-range organic eggs, preferably from small farms. To avoid salmonella food poisoning, cook until the yolk is firm and don't eat raw eggs – this means avoiding some homemade and restaurant ice cream, chocolate mousse and mayonnaise.

Meat Buy organic to be assured of meat free from hormones, pesticides and additives. Organic farms tend to reduce stock densities, with the result that animal husbandry is more humane and animals suffer less infection (and so require fewer antibiotics). This is particularly true of chicken and pork. In America, ask your butcher for hormone-free meat. Organically reared beef fed on pastures and certified organic dried

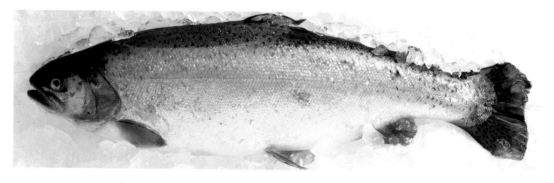

feed rather than processed feed potentially has less saturated fat and more good fats, such as omega-3 fatty acids and conjugated linoleic acid. Organic meat often has a firmer texture and better flavour because of the fat content (if this worries you, cut it off on the plate). Game such as pheasant, quail and rabbit is likely to be healthily free-range.

When not buying organic, choose traditional breeds raised on named farms and seek out a knowledgeable butcher to guide you. In supermarkets, ask whether routine antibiotics and growth promoters are permitted in the diet of chicken, beef, lamb and pork. Some advise trimming off the fat of non-organic meat and removing skin from poultry, the parts of the animal in which chemicals accrue.

Organic sausages and other processed meat products are prepared without the full range of chemicals allowed in conventional processing and run less risk of pesticide residue and antibiotics. Look out also for local quality specialities with limited ingredients: supermarket sausages may contain up to 15 non-food additives.

Meat to avoid: Raw and rare-cooked meat, including seared steaks and Parma ham; it carries the risk of toxoplasmosis which can cause brain damage and blindness in developing babies. Avoid also unpasteurized and non-UHT patés, which may carry the Listeria bug. Liver and its paté should also be given a miss. Intensive farming has led to very high levels of retinol in liver, with an associated risk of birth defects.

Fats

Some fats are essential during pregnancy for energy, vitamin absorption and a healthy nervous system. Maximize your daily quota of 8 percent of your food intake (2-3 portions a day) by choosing monounsaturated and polyunsaturated oils rich in omega-6 or omega-3 fatty acids. The latter are critical for fetal brain and eye development and vascular health. These good oils also help your milk production, reduce your risk of high blood pressure and premature delivery, and boost the baby's birthweight.

Monounsaturated fats Good sources are olive and rapeseed oils, nuts and avocados.

Polyunsaturated fats
Omega-6 oils from sunflower and sesame seeds and oils, safflower and corn oil. Omega-3 oils from oily fish, particularly mackerel; linseed and hemp oils; almonds, walnuts and cashew nuts; pumpkin seeds, sweet potato.

Low-tox sources
Substitute a little organic butter for processed margarines. Organic oils are cold-pressed at low temperatures which preserves maximum nutrients. Favour those in glass bottles. Hemp oil does not need to be grown with pesticides, and so is unlikely to be tainted with chemical residues. Non-organic safflower oil may contain lindane residues; soybean oil traces of dieldrin. Organic nuts and seeds won't be coated with petrol-based oils or sulphur dioxide – always buy organic sesame seeds and cashews. If you have a family history of asthma, eczema, food allergies or hay fever, avoid peanuts during pregnancy, and for extra peace of mind, sesame seeds, too.

Psst... **Vitamin supplements** Many pregnant women like to take a pregnancy multivitamin as a prenatal insurance policy. Some nutritionists believe that, apart from folic acid and perhaps iron, supplements are unnecessary if you eat a well-balanced diet and have no specific health needs. Supplements may even be potentially harmful: doses are unregulated, there are no standards for what goes into them, and their ability to harm a fetus is underevaluated, say some toxicologists. Reassuringly, eating plenty of fresh organic fruit, vegetables and high-quality meat gives you a range of ingredients that work synergistically – the blend of antioxidants, phyto-chemicals and other components creates a health effect more powerful than the individual ingredients alone.

Top pregnancy foods

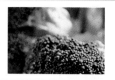

Broccoli For folate, calcium and antioxidant vitamins A, C and E. Stimulates the body's detox systems. Vitamin A is especially important in the first trimester.

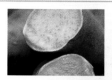

Sweet potatoes For vitamin C and folate, fibre and carbs. Choose deep red fleshed varieties for higher amounts of nasty-zapping beta-carotene (it also protects skin from sun damage). Eat with cereals to double iron absorption.

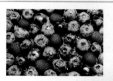

Berries Raspberries and blackberries, blueberries and cherries are rich in folate, vitamin C and phytonutrients (such as anthocyanin and ellagic and phenolic acid) that are strongly antioxidant.

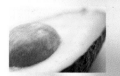

Avocados Rich in folate, vitamins B6, C and E, potassium, monounsaturated fats and antioxidant alpha-carotene. Folate offers up to 70 percent protection against defects to a baby's neural tube.

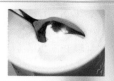

Natural yogurt More calcium than milk (a quarter of your daily requirement in one pot). Also high in zinc, protein and even fibre. Calcium is especially important between weeks 4 and 6.

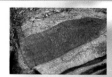

Organic beef The choice for B vitamins, highly absorbable iron, zinc, and of course, protein. One of the richest sources of choline. Zinc protects against low birthweight and birth defects.

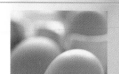

Eggs Packed with minerals and more than 12 vitamins. The chromium in the yolk can ward off first trimester nausea.

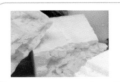

Hard cheese Good eating for calcium and vitamin B12, protein, fat and carbs. B12 safeguards a baby's developing brain and nervous system.

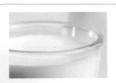

Milk All the qualities of cheese but with vitamin D and extra Bs. A bottle of organic a day contains your entire daily recommended intake of omega-3 fatty acid. If you can't get organic, semi-skimmed has almost as much calcium as full fat.

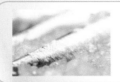

Oily fish Small fish, such as herring, mackerel and organic or wild salmon, are the best source of brain-boosting omega-3 fatty acids. They also contain valuable amounts of iron, calcium and zinc, B and D vitamins and protein.

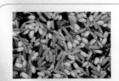

Wholegrains The real thing: with the bran and germ come fibre and nutrients stripped out in the refining process, including the antioxidant lignan and others necessary for healthy gut flora. Always choose organic.

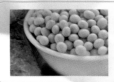

Chick peas Contain the antioxidant and immune-stimulant saponin as well as folate, fibre, iron and essential protein for vegetarians. Eat with a source of vitamin C for maximum absorption of iron.

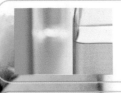

Olive oil Rich in antioxidant phenolics and vitamin E as well as oleic acid to boost the development of an unborn baby's brain and nervous system.

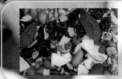

Seeds and nuts Packed with the nutrients needed to nurture germination and new life, they include antioxidant ellagic acid and lignans, selenium, magnesium and vitamin E, protective phytic acid, plus omega-3 fats to boost brain development.

How to eat and drink

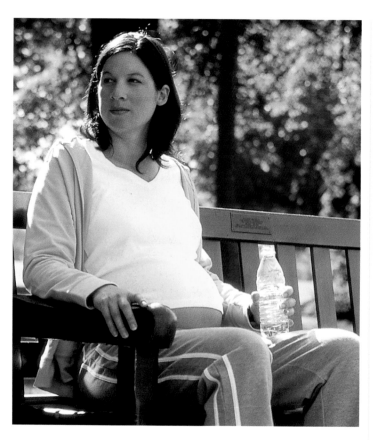

Great combinations

The greater the variety of foods you eat a little of each day, the more likely you (and your baby) will be well nourished. Food gets more nutritious when combined well, research shows. Certain vegetables eaten together, for instance, have more benefits than when consumed singly – mushrooms and broccoli work to inhibit cancer better together than alone; orange juice and oats are more artery-friendly in combination, and orange juice with dried apricots better for iron absorption.

Combine differently coloured foods on your plate: deep green, red or orange and yellow foods contain differing levels of healthy plant nutrients. Eat fresh fruit and vegetables with a source of fat (think salads with a slug of extra-virgin olive oil) to better absorb fat-soluble nutrients. Bring together vitamin-filled vegetables with wholegrains, meat and fish, and healthy fats at most mealtimes. Fit in raw fruit and vegetables in between for maximum nutrients and steam other vegetables briefly just before serving to reserve goodness.

The days of missing meals, especially breakfast, and of turning down snacks between meals are over. You may find now that you need to graze through the day to stave off nausea and suit a stomach shifted out of place by an important visitor. Try five or six nutrient-rich smaller meals. Eat like the Mediterraneans – slowly, sitting at a table with the TV off, savouring every mouthful (good posture and focusing on the food reduces the risk of indigestion). Put down your knife and fork between bites; have a conversation while you eat, and let the enjoyment of taste and texture be a de-stressing break in your day. Valuing food and making mealtimes special makes every day a little less toxic. One thing that is off the menu, however, is alcohol. The latest findings support find that there is no such thing as a safe level of alcohol during pregnancy. Miscarriage, low birthweight, reduced cognitive development, behavioural problems and FAS (fetal alcohol syndrome) are all risks associated with drinking during pregnancy.

Good hydration

Keeping well hydrated is vital for all that extra blood circulating in your body, working hard to deliver the nutrients that keep you and your baby healthy. It also helps your brain functioning: brain signals are transmitted more effectively in a watery environment. Drinking water helps prevent constipation and flushes out bacteria that may cause pregnancy urinary tract infections, while plumping up your skin from the inside out.

Aim for 6-8 glasses (approximately 2L a day). If pure water makes you feel nauseous, try carbonated versions with a squeeze of lime juice or make up your daily quota with milk, fresh-pressed fruit juices (dilute with water to ward off sugar rushes) and safe herbal teas (see page 20).

Caffeine

Many women first sense they might be pregnant because they go off tea and coffee. This may be nature hinting that the caffeine in these beverages isn't so good during pregnancy: imbibing large quantities has been associated with miscarriage. It also can cause insomnia and headaches, and drinking it within an hour of eating interferes with take-up of iron and folic acid. Caffeine has a diuretic effect, and so tea, coffee, cola, and to a lesser extent, chocolate drinks could leave you dehydrated. Stick to less than three mugs of coffee a day (make them milky lattes), six of tea or cocoa, or eight cans of cola if you must. Accompany with a glass of water. Decaffeinated coffee may contain traces of methylene chloride, which is carcinogenic (look for non solvent-extracted products).

"Sugar-free" drinks

In many soft drinks branded "sugar-free" or "diet", the sugar content has been replaced with aspartame or saccharin, best avoided in pregnancy.

Also avoid carbonated drinks that may contain additives such as the yellow food colouring tartrazine linked with growth retardation and hyperactivity in children as well as headaches and allergic reactions.

How to feel safer with your water

* Find out what's in your water. Contact your water company. You could have a sample of tap water tested by mail for contaminants, such as lead and copper, in pipes and taps old and new. (Try your supplier or Yellow Pages under Labs). If your water comes from a well have it tested yearly for heavy metals, nitrates, pesticides and bacteria. Be aware that farmers' springtime spraying can cause peaks in contamination levels.
* Run taps for 1-2 minutes before drawing water, especially first thing in the morning to flush through water that has been sitting in pipes overnight.
* Filter drinking water. The cheapest way is in a jug filter (change the cartridge regularly) or a kettle with built-in filter. Systems such as Pur and Brita remove lead, copper, chlorine and zinc, but don't generally touch nitrates, sulphates, some pathogens and pesticides. Under-the-sink reverse-osmosis systems bring triple-filtered water through your tap. They remove all the chemicals above, plus arsenic, cadmium, many pesticides, nitrates, sulphates and radium, but not all DBPs. Systems are relatively expensive to install. Worktop-standing water distillation systems remove all the above but not most pesticides, chlorine, or DBPs. They can be expensive and involve a lengthy wait for strange-tasting water depleted of useful calcium and magnesium. And tap water in lab tests had higher levels of bisphenol-A once purified!

Real food made easy

Food can be frightening when you're pregnant. If you don't want to worry about the food you eat, follow the suggestions below. Many of the foods are rich in antioxidant nutrients that help neutralize cell-damaging free-radicals produced by the body in response to pollution, stress and other toxins.

Sustaining breakfasts to avert nausea
- Homemade muesli of jumbo oats, assorted nuts and seeds, eaten with yogurt and fresh mango or melon.
- Berry smoothie with toasted nuts and seeds.
- Oat and milk porridge, with added chopped dried organic apricots sweetened with ginger syrup.
- Boiled eggs and toast.

Craving busters when ravenous
- Milky drink: organic cocoa is a powerful antioxidant.
- Banana or punnet of berries.
- Crudités: broccoli florets, slices of red pepper and carrots, celery sticks and cucumber, crunchy mangetout peas or handfuls of baby tomatoes.
- Pots of guacamole, humus and cottage cheese.
- Natural yogurt: sweeten with a drizzling of honey.

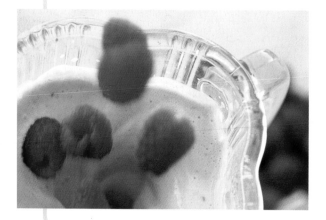

- Avocado: slice in half, add a splash of balsamic vinegar, and eat with a teaspoon.
- Chunks of hard cheese with a tasty organic apple – in season, look for russets and Coxes.
- Fresh sweetcorn in season, boiled, with a lick of butter.

Snacks for your handbag or desk drawer
- Bottle of water.
- Easy-to-peel organic satsumas.
- Oat cakes or crackers.
- Organic breadsticks.
- Tubs of assorted seeds – try sunflower, pumpkin, pine nuts and sesame seeds.
- Bags of almonds or Brazil nuts.
- Cartons of orange juice and milk.
- Organic carrots.
- Packs of sundried raisins.

Healthy lunches
- Crusty wholemeal bread with good hard cheeses and salad.
- Steak sandwich (well done) served with salad.
- Grilled fresh sardines served with a squeeze of lemon juice, olive oil, wholemeal bread and a salad.
- Beans on wholemeal toast with a grating of cheese.
- Tuna salad and a glass of milk.
- Bunches of watercress and baby spinach leaves with thin-sliced red pepper, slices of avocado, lightly steamed broccoli florets, halved baby tomatoes, toasted sunflower seeds and a dash of balsamic vinegar and olive oil.
- Smoked salmon bagel with cream cheese and a squeeze of lemon juice.
- Watercress soup with a little onion and potato.

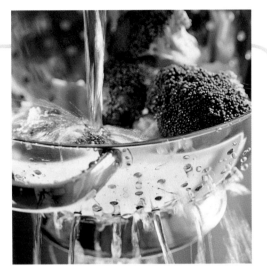

Instant suppers

- Cook double quantities and freeze your own ready meals low in saturated fat, salt and other additives. Major on nourishing soups and casseroles for healthy and almost effortless homecooked dishes.
- Roast an organic chicken or joint of free-range lamb or beef. Eat cold with fresh vegetables, salsas and salads the next day.
- Bake organic potatoes and serve with chicken, cheese and salads.
- Make an omelette, grating over a good helping of cheese.
- Poach salmon or hoki in milk or simply grill or pan-fry.
- Sweat leafy greens in a little olive oil with strips of red pepper, then mix into cooked pasta with toasted pine nuts and plenty of parmesan.
- Roast red pepper, whole tomatoes, onion and garlic, beetroot and carrot and serve on a bed of couscous with grilled halloumi cheese.
- Accompany sausages with a helping of lentils, prepared in advance.
- Stir-fry bean sprouts with seaweed, tofu, plenty of freshly sliced vegetables and a slug of walnut and sesame oil. Serve with noodles.

Sweet alternatives

- Homemade popcorn.
- 70 percent cocoa solid organic chocolate.
- Freshly made pancakes smeared with butter and a squeeze of lemon juice.
- Fruit scones served warm with good jam and clotted cream.
- Dried organic apricots, figs and prunes.
- Well-supplied (interesting) fruit bowl.
- Wholemeal seeded bread, toasted with butter and Marmite/jam/honey.
- Slow-cooked rice puddings.

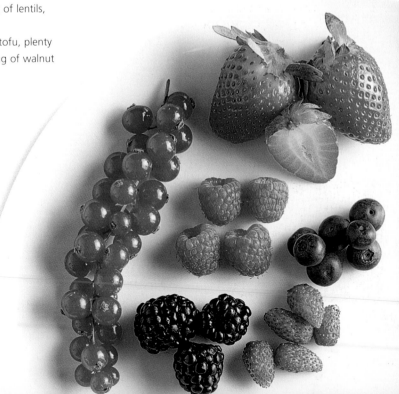

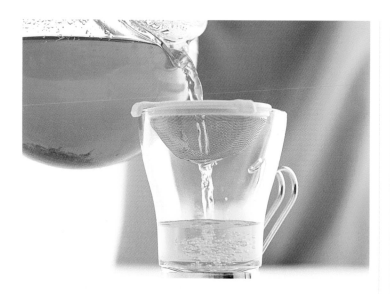

Herbal teas

Some herbs are uterine stimulants and can bring on contractions. The following should not be taken during pregnancy. Ginseng tea; brews containing cohash, slippery elm, pennyroyal and mugwort; fennel, liquorice and sage tea.

Peppermint tea Take as a digestif after dinner to replace your regular espresso, but don't drink to excess, as the herb is a potent uterine stimulant.

Ginger tea Grate a 2-inch section of fresh ginger root into a cup. Pour over boiling water and leave to steep for 10 minutes. Sweeten with honey and add a squeeze of fresh lemon juice for extra perkiness.

Camomile tea Although the essential oil is contraindicated during early pregnancy for its ability to stimulate the uterus, the tea, drunk in moderation, is gently relaxing. Don't have more than 1 cup a day if you've suffered spotting or a history of miscarriage.

Raspberry leaf tea The stalwart drink of natural birth advocates. Drink only during the final 6-8 weeks of pregnancy and during labour. For a more palatable brew, mix half in half with verbena tea.

Great juices

Press your own organic fruit juices. Farmers' markets often sell bags of misshapen or extremely ripe organic fruit cheaply.

- Apple and ginger juice makes a zingy pick-me-up.
- Blackthorn juice is celebrated for its fortifying and invigorating properties during "growth phases" such as pregnancy when you feel exhausted and jaded. Dilute with boiling water for a warming winter tonic. Weleda's

is made from certified organic ingredients collected from controlled wild sites.

- If you find it hard to wean yourself off carbonated soft drinks, try mixing fruit juice with sparkling water.
- For more of a meal, add yogurt and milk to juiced mango, kiwi, melon, and berries and whizz to create a nutritious smoothie.
- For parties mix non-alcoholic fruit cocktails – orange with a dash of cranberry; orange and grapefruit with a squeeze of lemon juice and plenty of ice; exotic medleys of pineapple, mango and coconut.

Psst... Phytochemicals

These are biologically active compounds found in all plant food of which there are hundreds. Their full range of benefits have yet to be discovered but among them are antioxidants, which make a valuable contribution to your general cell health. Other common phytochemicals are bioflavonoids, isoflavones, lignans, and phytoestrogens. Fruits and vegetables are filled with these valuable nutrients and juices are an easy way to get your fill.

Reducing your risk

- Shop at greengrocers and markets where items are available loose and wrapped in paper bags.
- Carry a cloth bag or basket so you don't have to load your home (and garbage) with plastic bags.
- In the supermarket, choose items with less layers of packaging.
- Select drinks in glass bottles, especially milk and juices.
- Avoid plastic packaging marked with a 3 in a triangle; it's made from PVC.
- Where possible, choose unbleached paper or halogen-free plastic packaging.
- Write to your supermarket requesting their policies on packaging. Ask whether they have plans to phase out PVC or replace plastic foam containers with paper.
- Don't reuse plastic packaging from one product for another type of product. Manufacturers only have to ensure a package is safe for the food it originally contains.
- Avoid dishwashing, boiling or brushing plastic or wrap containing bisphenol-A, which can cause it to migrate into food. Dishwasher-safe plastic containers are marked.
- Be especially careful when wrapping "wet" products containing a good proportion of fat, acid or alcohol in plastic. One study shows that if an acidic food, such as a peeled orange, is wrapped in a plastic bread bag turned inside out, in 10 minutes the fruit could absorb 5 percent of the lead in the printing ink. Eating 2-3 oranges would provide a dose of lead potent enough to observe toxic effects in a fetus.

- Don't reuse plastic water bottles for juice or milk.
- Only use microwave plastic containers marked "microwave safe". Some people prefer to transfer frozen foods to ceramic or Pyrex dishes before heating.
- Don't use clingfilm where it might melt (e.g. in conventional ovens).
- Make sure clingfilm doesn't touch food in a microwave, risking migration of chemicals into food.
- Only use clingfilm on high-fat foods, such as cheese, fatty meats, pastries and topped cakes where the manufacturer states it is safe to use clingfilm.
- Don't store ingredients in opened cans in the fridge, which may expose foods to lead.

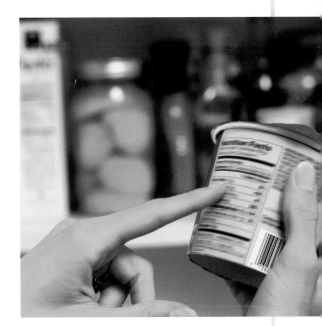

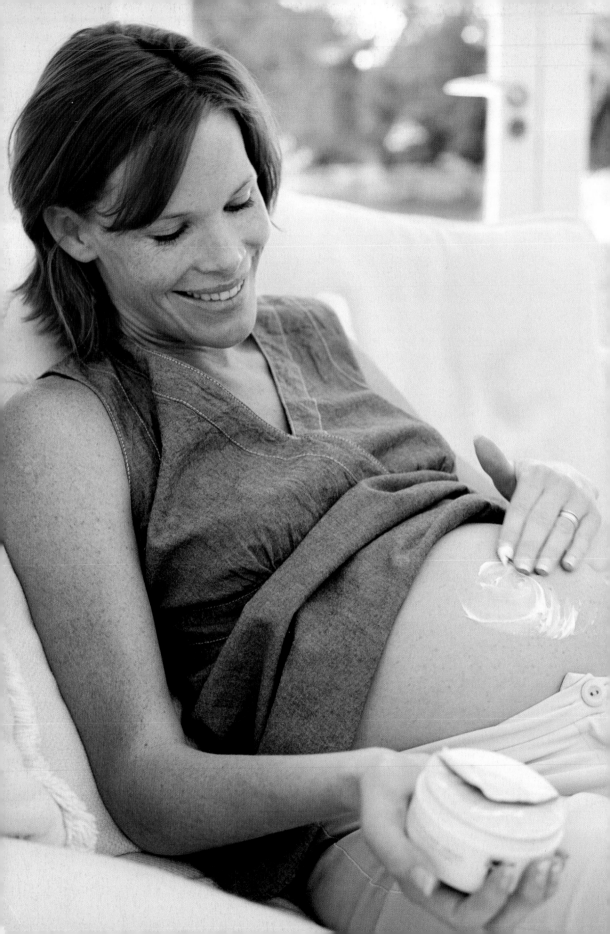

Skin, hair & tooth care

If you care about what you eat during pregnancy, then you should care about what you use on your body, since 60 percent of what we apply to the skin, from body lotions to antiperspirants, is absorbed; 80 percent when the skin is wet. When you're pregnant and trying to minimize your exposure to potentially noxious substances by eating organic food and using water-based DIY products, you need to be reassured that what you put on your skin, hair and teeth isn't potentially harmful to your health and the development of your baby. Unfortunately, many products sold on the high street contain potentially dangerous substances. That's why I show you how to prepare plenty of all-natural unguents that smell good, and feel satiny on the skin as well as those that will keep your hair and teeth in glowing health. By using chemical-free products you'll boost your self-confidence that you're doing everything you can to protect yourself and your growing baby.

Safe skincare

Here are safe, natural skincare solutions to combat everyday pregnancy skin problems using easy-to-make recipes concocted from the contents of your fridge. Such "food-grade" ingredients make perfect sense during pregnancy, when you shouldn't put on your skin anything you wouldn't eat. If you make up the products yourself, you can be sure the ingredients are fresh, organic and risk-free. Use them to replace makeup remover, notoriously chock-full of chemical nasties, especially impregnated wipes. These easy oils also pump beneficial vitamins and essential fatty acids into your bloodstream, which can only nourish your baby.

Daily routine

Mix up a cleanser and moisturizer to suit your skin type using the recipes opposite, then follow this cleanse, tone and moisturize regime.

1 Remove makeup by coating a cotton ball in the makeup remover. Wipe over your face. Remove excess oil by soaking a clean washcloth in warm water; squeeze well and wipe across the skin.
2 Massage the cleanser over your face and neck, paying attention to areas prone to breakouts. Fill a bowl with very warm water and add 2 tsp rosewater. Soak the washcloth in the solution. Squeeze out, then use to wipe away the cleanser. Rinse, squeeze out and repeat as often as feels good.
3 To tone and close pores, wipe the face with a cotton ball soaked in rosewater.
4 Pour a few drops of the moisturizing oil into the palm of one hand. Warm by rubbing your palms together, then pick up a little on your fingertips and massage into your face and neck using gentle upward strokes. Finish by gently circling at the temples with eyes closed for a few minutes, breathing in the scents of the essential oils.

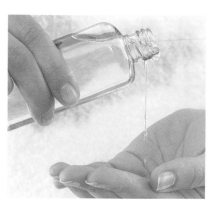

Natural cleansers

Simple to create, these gentle cleansers have been used for generations to draw out dirt and soothe sensitive skin. In all recipes, avoid nuts and their oils if allergic to nuts, wheatgerm oil if allergic to wheat, milk if allergic to dairy.

Gentle makeup remover

2 tbsp sweet almond or sunflower oil
2 drops essential oil of neroli
Pour the almond oil into a sterilized dark glass bottle. Drop in the essential oil, replace the lid and store in a cool dark place. Shake before use.

Dry skin cleanser

1 tsp fine oatmeal
1 tsp avocado oil
1 tsp milk powder
½ tsp runny honey
1-2 tbsp single cream
Blend together the oatmeal, oil and milk powder. Mix in the honey and cream to make a thick paste.

Sensitive skin cleanser

1 tsp fine oatmeal
1 tsp sweet almond oil
1 tsp milk powder
1-2 tbsp rosewater
Blend together the oatmeal, oil and milk powder. Mix in enough rosewater to make a smooth paste.

Oily skin cleanser

1 tsp ground almonds
1 tsp sweet almond or grapeseed oil

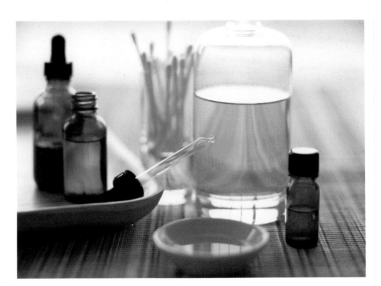

Pour the sunflower oil into a sterilized dark glass container. Prick the vitamin E capsule and squeeze in the contents. Drop in the essential oils and replace the lid.

Combination skin moisturizer

2 tbsp sweet almond or
   grapeseed oil
1 vitamin E capsule
2 drops essential oil of neroli
1 drop essential oil of ylang ylang
Pour the sweet almond oil into a sterilized dark glass container. Prick the vitamin E capsule and squeeze in the contents. Drop in the essential oils and replace the lid.

1 tsp finely grated zest of 1 lime
1-2 tbsp orange blossom water
Blend together the almond powder, oil and lime zest. Mix in enough orange blossom water to make a thin paste.

Combination skin cleanser

1 camomile tea bag
1 tsp ground almonds
1 tsp sweet almond or grapeseed
   oil
1 tsp milk powder
Place the tea bag in a mug and pour over boiling water. Steep for 20 minutes. Blend together the almond powder, oil and milk powder. Mix in enough camomile tea to make a smooth paste.

Natural moisturizers

These oils contain extracts of fruit, nuts and flowers gentle enough for use in pregnancy. Store in a cool dark place and shake before use.

Dry skin moisturizer

2 tbsp apricot kernel oil
1 tsp wheatgerm oil
2 drops essential oil of frankincense
1 drop essential oil of rosewood
Pour the apricot and wheatgerm oils into a sterilized dark glass container. Drop in the essential oils and replace the lid.

Sensitive skin moisturizer

2 tbsp peach kernel oil
1 vitamin E capsule
3 drops essential oil of sandalwood
Pour the peach oil into a sterilized dark glass container. Prick the capsule and squeeze in the contents. Drop in the essential oil and replace the lid.

Oily skin moisturizer

2 tbsp sunflower oil
1 vitamin E capsule
2 drops essential oil of petitgrain
1 drop essential oil of palmarosa

Psst... **Itchy skin?**
When you switch from beauty products based on petrol derivatives to plant oils, you may find your skin suffers from dryness, itching and peeling. Don't give up immediately. Natural beauty therapists regard this as a period of adjustment from the skin's addiction to petrol-derived oils that cake the skin – see it as a mini detox. Living Nature advise you wait a week for your skin to restore some natural balance; The Organic Pharmacy urges you to allow one month for skin to adjust.

Deep cleansing routine

Use this routine with its accompanying recipes (see right), once a week to prevent blackheads and calm irritated skin. The green tea toner, recommended for its soothing properties, may relieve acne and has also been shown to protect skin from the ageing effects of exposure to ultraviolet light and environmental toxins. The yogurt in the softening mask is a natural exfoliant (its lactic acid shifts dead cells from the skin's surface, encouraging the process of cell renewal).

1 Cleanse the face and neck using your regular routine and everyday cleansing products (see pages 24-25).
2 Massage the scrub into your face and neck, paying attention to the side of the nose, where pores often get blocked, and other sites of spots, such as the chin and forehead. Soak a washcloth in warm water, squeeze, then wipe away the scrub. Repeat until every trace is gone.
3 Tone by soaking cotton balls in the cooled green tea, and wiping them over the face to remove traces of cleanser.
4 Smooth the fruit mask onto your face and neck, avoiding the eye area. Place the chilled green tea bags (or peeled, sliced potato) on your eyes and a chilled eye mask on top, if desired. Wrap yourself in a blanket and recline on pillows for 10 minutes. Try to erase all thoughts from your mind.
5 Soak a washcloth in warm water, wring out, then wipe away the mask. Repeat as many times as needed to cleanse face and neck. Repeat the green tea toning. Then moisturize with the facial oil using the facelifting strokes of facial massage (see page 27).

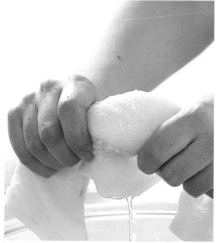

Deep cleansers

Gentle scrub

2 tsp fine oatmeal
2 tsp milk powder
½ teaspoon sunflower oil
1 tbsp rosewater

Mix together the oatmeal and milk powder, then stir in the oil to make a thick paste. Let down with as much rosewater as required to create the consistency you prefer.

Green tea toner

Place 2 green tea bags in separate mugs. Pour over boiling water and leave to cool. Once cool, remove the bags and refrigerate. Reserve the tea.

Banana avocado mask

1 very ripe banana
1 very ripe avocado
1-2 tbsp thick natural yogurt
1 tbsp runny honey

Peel the fruit and mash the flesh. When you have the consistency you prefer, stir in the yogurt and honey.

Grapeseed moisturizing oil

1 vitamin E capsule
2 tbsp grapeseed oil
1 drop each essential oils of
    sandalwood and frankincense

Prick the vitamin capsule and squeeze the contents into the grapeseed oil. Mix in the essential oils well.

Facial massage

This reviving facial self-massage will lift tension and encourage lightness and softness back into the face, giving the impression of a facelift. Grapeseed is a powerful antioxidant capable of protecting the skin against the premature ageing triggered by toxins such as cigarette and exhaust smoke.

1 Apply a little of the grapeseed moisturizing oil to your fingertips and rub your palms together to warm and distribute the oil. Apply more oil as necessary during the massage to keep your movements flowing.

2 Turning your head to the right, place the backs of your hands where your neck meets your shoulder. Using alternate hands, stroke the backs of your fingers up to the jaw in a seamless stroking action. Turn your head to the left and repeat on the right side of the neck.

3 Pinch the chin between your index fingers and thumbs and sweep them out along the jawline to the ears several times. Then make circular pressures with your thumbs at the angle of the jaw, where many people hold tension.

4 Massage all around the ears, rolling and circling them between your fingers and thumbs.

5 Repeat the repetitive stroking movement with the backs of the fingers of alternate hands up from your jaw over your left cheek. Repeat over the right cheek.

6 Place your middle fingers at the sides of your mouth and make tiny circles all around the mouth, working quite deeply. Press and hold for a moment at the sides of the mouth, in the chin dimple, and above the cupid's bow.

7 Place your ring fingers where your eyebrows meet the bridge of your nose. Sweep out over the eyebrow around the eye socket and gently down over the cheekbones beneath the eyes and up to your starting position. Build up a seamless flow of strokes. Then tap your fingertips very lightly out from where the cheekbones join your nose to your temples to relieve puffiness.

8 With thumbs and index fingers, pinch the eyebrows from the centre out: squeeze, release and move outward to repeat.

9 Rest the fingertips of both hands at the centre of your forehead. Draw outward to your temples several times, circling your index fingers at the temples each time.

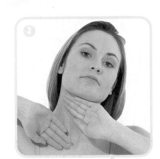

10 Place your index fingers in the centre of your forehead and criss-cross them in a scissor-like action, as if erasing frown lines. Repeat out to the left and right.

11 Roll the length of alternate index fingers up over your forehead from eyebrows to hairline. Repeat from left to right.

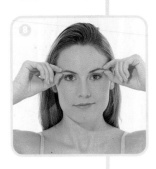

12 To finish, rest your palms over your face (don't put pressure on the eye balls) for a few moments, opening your eyes to look into the darkness of your palms. Draw your hands outward.

Blending body oils at home

Pure nut and seed oils smooth the skin so effectively and are so healthy and cheap to buy that you might like to blend your own. Experiment with some of these good options for pregnancy. Choose organic cold-pressed oils where possible, using the base oils on their own or blending in one or more of the speciality enriching oils.
Caution: Do a patch test, especially if you are allergic to nuts or wheat, by rubbing a little of the oil you plan to use in the inside of your wrist. If no reaction occurs within 24 hours, it's safe to use that oil.

Base oils

Extra-virgin olive oil Full of skin-protecting vitamin E, minerals, fatty acids and oleic acid (vital for bone growth) and a little protein. A

fantastic moisturizer, it is said to rejuvenate cells and is ideal for very dry or inflamed skin. It's well absorbed into the skin, if a little sticky.

Sweet almond oil A very light oil full of vitamins – A, B1, B2, E, F – that's soothing for dry, sensitive skin, especially for eczema and chapped hands. Doesn't absorb instantly so better for massage than as a morning body oil.

Apricot kernel oil Another oil for delicate skin rich in minerals and vitamins, including A, B1, B2 and B6. Easily absorbed.

Sunflower seed oil Best for very delicate skin and has a light fragrance that won't disturb sensitized noses. Contains the essential fatty acid linoleic acid, minerals and vitamins A, B, D and E. Light in texture and easily absorbed.

Grapeseed oil Contains a high concentration of cell membrane-strengthening polyphenols that protect elastin and collagen fibres, and are 10,000 times more powerful than vitamin E at neutralizing skin-damaging free radicals. A good all-rounder.

Enriching oils

Sesame seed oil Lightweight oil especially suitable for dry skin, with a good supply of vitamins and minerals and a little protein has UV light-filtering properties and soothes sunburnt skin.

Avocado oil Contains restorative vitamins A, E and D and suits very dry skin and eczema.

Jojoba Rich but light-textured liquid wax from a bean that's good for irritated scalps and very dry skin since it resembles the chemical structure of the skin and hair's natural lubricant, sebum. A source of antioxidant vitamin E, valued for its regenerative properties. Suits allergic skin and acne, too. Waxy and easily absorbed for those who dislike the greasiness of oils, it leaves a protective barrier on skin to reduce moisture loss. Shown to increase skin softness by more than 35 percent. Use to thicken blends and prevent spoiling.

Hemp oil Source of vital omega fats -3, -6 and -9. Thought to be helpful with eczema. Use it on salads, too: natural beauty therapists say after two weeks you'll notice softer skin.

Macadamia oil Nice nutty-scented oil rich in protein, vitamins and the

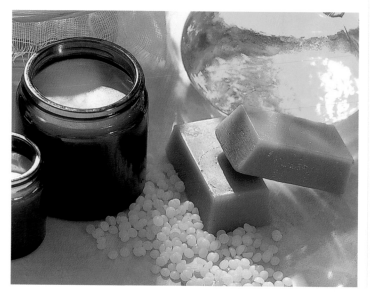

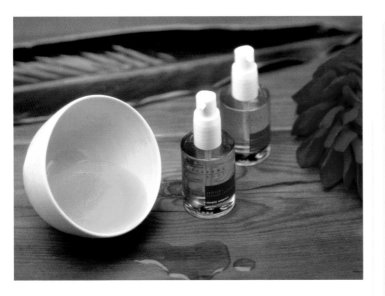

minerals selenium, zinc and potassium.

Rosehip oil Very good for skin thanks to high levels of fatty acids. Renowned for rejuvenating and repairing scarred and sun-damaged skin and repairing chemically damaged hair. Advised for use pre-surgery: rub into your belly for two weeks before a planned caesarean.

Wheatgerm oil Very rich in vitamin E. Add a few drops to a blend to prevent rancidity. Can speed the healing of sunburn and scar tissue; you might like to include it in your birthing bag.

Off-the-shelf alternatives

Cleansers

For dry, delicate skin look for emollient cleansers, such as Living Nature's Vitalizing Creamy Cleanser, based on nut and olive oils and honey. For removing makeup at night try Weleda's Almond Facial Oil, blended from sweet almond, plum and blackthorn extracts, and soothing both for cleansing and nighttime regeneration.

Facial oils

Many facial moisturizers created from organic oils, beeswax, essential oils and other macerated botanicals are oil-based and don't work so well under makeup. Reserve these oils and serums for nighttime. The Organic Pharmacy recommends holding creams at night to allow the skin to breathe and go about its natural cleansing and elimination processes. Living Nature's Balancing Epo and Honey Night Gel is good even for eczema-prone skin, or choose REN's superb Omega-3 Oil.

Facial creams

When skin is super-sensitive (and nose extra-sensitive to perfume), choose Weleda's Almond Skincare range, free of essential oils but almond-scented. The creamy Moisture Cream is ultra-light for daywear.

Lip softeners

Pregnancy dry skin can extend to dry lips, which worsen when a stuffy noses keeps you breathing through your mouth. The condition can be exacerbated by swimming,

air conditioning and long-last lipsticks. Instead of a petroleum-based product, try Jurlique's Lip Care Balm made from safflower oil, shea and cocoa butters, beeswax and oils from the castor and jojoba plants and macadamia nut. Green People's No Scent Soft Lips combines shea butter (which can help shield from UV radiation) with organic aloe vera.

Eye gels

To firm puffy skin, look for products based on plant proteins, such as Green People's Eye Gel, Living Nature's Firming Eye Gel, or The Organic Pharmacy's Lip and Eye Cream.

Hand treatments

You can continue to keep your hands looking great using natural and home-made products. Below, and on the following pages, you will find treatments and products that promote good health and are free of dangerous chemicals.

Step-by-step manicure

1 Remove old nail polish with an acetone-free remover. Do it outside, or at the least open a window to help ventilation, then soak a cotton ball in the remover and sweep from cuticle to tip. You may need to use several balls to remove dark colours.

2 Sit back and relax for 10-15 minutes as you soften hands and nails by plunging them into a nail bath (choose from the recipes on page 32). Use a nailbrush if necessary to clean away dirt. Pat dry with a warm fluffy towel.

3 Carefully ease out dirt from beneath each nail using a cotton bud.

4 Wrap another cotton ball around the tip of an orange stick and dip into a little avocado oil. Gently ease the cuticles back from each nail.

5 File nails with a long emery board, starting with the little finger of the right hand (or left hand if left-handed) and working inward. Make long strokes in one direction, working in from the outer edges. Use the more textured side first to reduce the length of the nail; finish with the finer surface. For a natural look, shape nails into a rounded oval. To strengthen brittle nails, straighten the tip to a blunt edge.

6 Cover your hands in a clay mask (see page 32), then raise your feet and close your eyes, relaxing for 10 minutes while the mask dries.

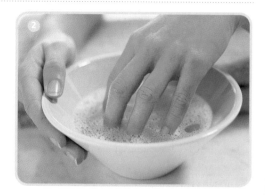

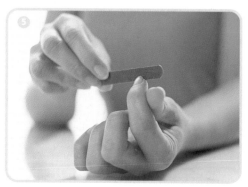

7 Rinse your hands in the nailbath and pat dry well. Buff nails to a high shine with a chamois (buffing stimulates circulation to the tips, bringing nutrients to the area to leave the nails naturally healthy). Follow with the self-massage sequence opposite.

Self-massage for the hands

This boosts circulation to the nails to keep them pink and healthy (buffing with a chamois has the same effect).

1 Bring circulation to the region by circling your hands at the wrist. Work slowly at first, circling outward without moving your forearms. Make the rotations slow and as wide as possible. Repeat in the other direction. Clench your knuckles, then flick out your fingers several times. Shake your hands loosely.

2 Pour a little of one of the moisturizing oils (see page 32) into one palm and rub your palms together to distribute the oil and warm your hands. Interlink your fingers and rub the webs of your fingers together.

3 Supporting the palm of one hand with the fingers of the other hand (rest the back of your supporting hand on your thigh), circle the middle of the palm with your thumb. Take the circle wider to cover the entire palm.

4 Massage the thumb and fingers from base to tip using the same circular stroke with your thumb and circling around the knuckles. Then use your working thumb

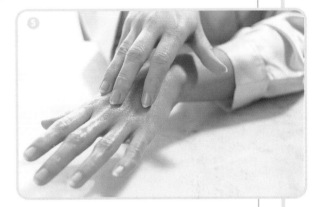

and index finger like a corkscrew up the digit. Squeeze at the tip as you pull your fingers away.

5 Turn the hand over, add a little more oil and slide your fingertips from the base of the fingers toward the wrist, working along each channel. Repeat.

6 Repeat steps 3-5 on the other hand. Interlink your fingers again, rubbing the webs, then palms together.

7 Finally, rub a little oil into each nail, squeezing each one so a little nourishing oil slips into the gap between nail and cuticle.

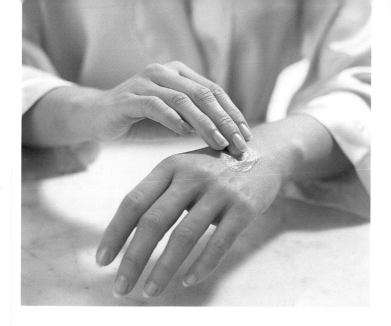

Natural nail baths

Cleansing bath Into a bowl of warm water, add a good squeeze of lemon juice.

Softening soak In a large bowl mix 1 tsp avocado oil into 6 tbsp milk powder. Add enough cool water to make a paste, stirring well to eliminate lumps, then top up with warm water, stirring constantly. (Avoid if allergic to milk.)

Conditioning bath Into a bowl of warm water, add 1 tsp olive oil, 2 tbsp orange flower water and 2 drops essential oil of benzoin.

Bath for very dry nails Into 2 tsp jojoba, squeeze the contents of 1 vitamin E capsule. Pour into a bowl of tepid water and swish until dispersed.

Homemade hand and nail moisturizers

Night treatment for chapped skin Mix 1 tbsp olive oil into 1 tbsp runny honey. Soak your hands in warm water, pat dry, then massage the honey oil mixture into hands, wrists and nails, put on cotton gloves and go to bed. By the morning your skin will be silky and your nails shining.

Clay mask for dry skin Into 2 tbsp kaolin (from pharmacies), mix enough rose water to make a smooth paste. Apply to the hands, relax for 10 minutes while the clay dries, then rinse off by plunging hands into a nail bath (see above).

Daily moisturizing oil Mix together 2 tbsp grapeseed oil and 1 tsp wheatgerm or rosehop oil. Squeeze in the contents of 1 vitamin E capsule and add 1 drop each essential oils of sandalwood and patchouli. Massage into the hands as needed, especially after washing up or washing hands.

Brittle nail oil Massage with 1 tsp olive oil mixed with ½ tsp rosehip oil and 1 drop essential oil of sandalwood.

Cuticle-conditioning oil Into 1 tsp sweet almond or olive oil, blend 1 drop essential oil of patchouli.

Off-the-shelf natural handcare

For dry, chapped hands

Green People's Dry Zone dry skin salve is a water-free light barrier cream made from almond, calendula and beeswax that's good for gardeners, too. Raid the baby's armoury for an intense, carroty-scented Baby's Soothing Cream from Jurlique, rich in calendula to restore skin that's inflamed, cracked, or allergy-prone.

To keep by the wash basin

Living Nature's Manuka Honey Hand and Body Cream blended from macadamia, avocado and wheatgerm oils suits even eczema-prone skin. Longlasting, it doubles as a foot balm.

Psst... Reading labels
This can be a tricky task. Some ingredients listings are sealed in packaging and can't be browsed until after you've bought. And not everything may appear on the label. The ingredients that make up fragrance/parfum are notoriously tricky: to safeguard commercial secrets, they don't have to be listed and this is where some of the more dubious chemicals for health are concentrated. Many ingredients listings use only the biological name, requiring you to become conversant in chemistry and Latin to be able to decipher common and often innocuous ingredients, such as honey or olive oil.

Foot treatments

Homemade scrub, oil and exfoliator

Sea salt scrub Into 1 tbsp fine sea salt, stir 1 tbsp runny honey, 1 tsp olive oil and 1 inch grated fresh ginger root. Massage into dry feet, especially around hard skin on the heels and balls of the feet. Rinse away in a foot bath.

Lemon and ginger massage oil Into 2 tbsp olive oil, blend 1 drop each essential oils of ginger and lemon. If you have sensitive skin, patch test the essential oils.

Fruity exfoliator Cut two pomegranates in half and scoop out the seeds. Rub the seed-laden flesh over your feet, then wrap each foot in an old warmed towel. Relax for 10 minutes before rinsing in a foot bath.

Off-the-shelf natural footcare

Foot balms

Weleda's Foot Balm has a cooling effect and great fresh scent. It's non-greasy. Jurlique's Foot and Leg Lotion is recommended at the beginning and end of the day. Spiezia Organics Organic Foot Balm has an intensely unguent consistency that requires only a tiny amount for lasting softness and new vitality when your feet are sore or tired. So natural it's edible, Burt's Bees Coconut Foot Crème brings together a surprisingly good fragrance of coconut and peppermint (to reduce puffiness). It also contains oat proteins to

exfoliate dry skin. Smother feet at night, put on cotton socks and retire to bed.

Non-toxic remedies for foot problems

As your bump gets bigger, your legs and feet have to support more weight. And as your posture shifts to accommodate the bump, so it can exacerbate or even cause lower back problems. Wearing heels that tip the pelvis forward only exaggerates the kink in the lower back, making problems worse. Postural aches and pains are even more miserable when retained moisture makes your feet puffy, too. Here are some natural solutions.

Aching legs and feet

Fashion cure Choose flatties for everyday wear, better for your posture and more stable when pregnancy clumsiness can cause falls. In the summer (and winter with a pair of chunky socks), no pregnant women should turn down the opportunity to look like a cool earth mother in Birkenstock sandals, which supply excellent support. For exercise, treat yourself to a pair of sneakers in your new size to help you maintain motivation and bring a bounce back into your step.

Massage cure From the second trimester onward use a heavyweight "green" foot moisturizer or massage oil morning and night for massage to relieve aches and revitalize.

Bath cure To a warm water footbath (in a bucket to soothe the calves, too), add 2 drops essential oil of orange or petitgrain and submerge the legs for up to 20 minutes.

Swollen ankles

By the third trimester the ankles often swell, a sign that you need to stop running around and start tending to your own needs.

Massage cure Follow the foot massage (see page 35) with smooth, gentle strokes up the calf and shin from ankle to knee.

Postural cure Practise ankle rotations when sitting motionless at a desk. Try keeping your legs elevated on a cushion.

Bath cure To a tepid water footbath, add 2 drops essential oil of bergamot and relax for up to 20 minutes. For hot, swollen feet make it a cool water footbath and add 2 drops essential oil of grapefruit. If you're really perspiring, throw in a few ice cubes. For itchy (or dry) feet, add 2 tsp jojoba to the water, swishing well to disperse.

Herbal cure Sip nettle tea (cover 1 tea bag with boiling water and leave to steep until cool enough to drink) for its diuretic effect.

Pedicure & foot massage

A pedicure is the ultimate luxury when you can no longer see your feet. Pregnancy is hard on the feet and the folllowing totally natural treatments may help to reduce the swellling a little, ease aches and pains and can add moisture to brittle nails.

Step-by-step pedicure

1 Open a window to aid ventilation, then remove old nail polish by soaking a cotton ball in acetone-free nail polish remover and sweeping from cuticle to tip.

2 Sit back and relax, cushioning the back of your waist to prevent lower-back ache. Plunge your feet into a bucket of warm water containing one of the footbath ideas on page 33. For an extra treat, throw in a wooden foot roller (available from pharmacies and natural health stores). Place it on the bottom of the footbath and roll the soles of your feet over it, working well over areas that feel sore. Relax reading a book or listening to music for 10 minutes. Sip a glass of water. If your toenails are dirty, scrub with a nail brush.

3 Dry toes well with a warmed fluffy towel. When absolutely dry, file nails with an emery board, making long strokes in one direction only, working in from the outer edges. Keep the tips flat.

4 Wrap a cotton ball around an orange stick and carefully ease the cuticles back from each nail. Don't push too far.

5 To tackle dry skin, massage in the sea salt scrub (see page 33) rubbing well around the heels and balls of the feet.

6 Rinse your feet in the footbath. Pat dry, paying attention to the often neglected area between the toes. Use a pumice stone to remove remaining dry skin, if necessary, sweeping in one direction only.

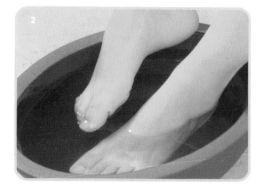

7 Make the fruity pomegranate exfoliator (see page 33) and rub the seed-laden flesh over your feet, paying special attention to areas of dry, hard skin. Wrap each foot in an old warmed towel, then raise your feet and relax for another 10 minutes.

8 Rinse feet again in the footbath and dry well. Buff nails with a chamois, then moisturize using the sequence of strokes opposite.

Foot massage

1 Bend one knee and bring the foot onto your opposite thigh if possible. If not, have someone else massage you. Pour a massage oil (see page 33) into one palm. Rub both palms together to spread and warm the oil. Sandwich the foot between your palms and glide your hands from ankle and heel to toes several times to spread the oil.

2 Sandwiching the toes between your hands, flex them toward the shin, then point them downward several times. Then, holding the foot, circle it, rotating at the ankle. Work in one direction, then the other, isolating the movement in the ankle joint by resisting movement in the lower leg.

3 Pointing the toes with one hand, run your other thumb along the grooves on the top of the foot from toe to ankle several times, then massage each toe between thumb and index finger, rotating and rubbing from base to tip and pressing firmly at the tip before pulling away.

4 Turn the foot so the sole is uppermost. Ripple your knuckles all over the sole, paying particular attention to areas that feel tense or tender. Wherever you feel tension, press into the sole with your knuckles firmly, turn the knuckles, release and move to repeat on another area of tension.

5 Supporting the top of your foot from beneath with the fingers of both hands, run your thumbs up the centre of the sole and out to the sides. Pull firmly outward, stretching the outer edges of the foot upward quite strongly. Hold for a few seconds before repeating the stroke several times.

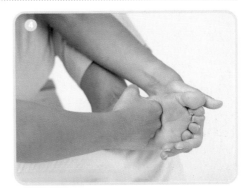

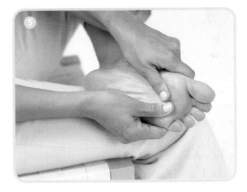

6 Inch up the sole from heel to toes, walking alternate thumbs like a caterpillar. Start at the instep, repeat down the centre of the sole, then along the outer edge.

7 Finish with more soothing sandwiching strokes along the length of the foot. Repeat all the strokes on the other foot.

8 Finally, rub a little extra oil into each nail, squeezing each one so nourishing oil slips into the gap between nail and cuticle. Wait 15 minutes for the oil to absorb, before slipping on cozy cashmere socks.

Sun protection

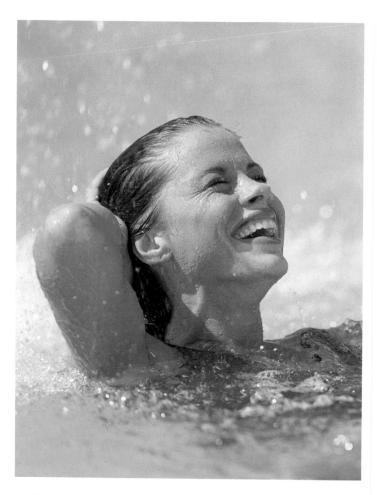

Off-the-shelf alternatives

Some ecocosmetic manufacturers refuse to make sunscreen, unconvinced they can create a produce that doesn't contain harmful substances. Most commercially available sunscreens contain PABA, chemical "sponges", are added to absorb ultraviolet rays, which have been found to be hormone disrupting and possibly linked to DNA damage.

Weleda's sunscreen contains no chemical sun filters, but it does contain titanium oxide and zinc oxide "micronized" into ultra-fine particles that don't tint the skin white.

Psst... Check your makeup If you're worried about exposing your skin to sunscreens, check the ingredients listing on your makeup. Moisturizer, lipstick and foundation may contain sunscreen to fulfil manufacturers' anti-wrinkle claims, since exposure to UV light produces premature ageing of the skin. Some natural beauticians state that sunscreens are unnecessary in nightcreams and products you use in winter, when you spend more time indoors and in the dark.

Wearing a sunscreen can make us feel so protected we stay in the sun longer than we would with bare skin, risking overheating as well as skin discoloration (in pregnancy we have higher levels of the hormone that produces the pigment melanin). Exposing yourself to UV light in this way can, of course, be a risk factor for skin cancer. Covering large expanses of the body with "leave-on" products also risks undesirable ingredients penetrating the skin.

However, some natural beauty advocates stress that a little sun exposure is even quite good for the body. Sunlight on skin promotes the formation of vitamin D, crucial for absorption of calcium, and particularly important for people with darker skins living in the northern hemisphere. Sunlight can also be effective in treating skin conditions, such as psoriasis, and it boosts immunity, which is lowered during pregnancy.

Until recently, titanium oxide/ dioxide were regarded as safer forms of sunscreen because they shield skin from both ultraviolet (UV) A and B rays by sitting in a layer on the surface (as in the white stripe beloved of surf dudes). They are also considered unlikely to cause allergic reactions or skin irritation. Now, smaller "nano" particles of the substance are being used that can penetrate the skin (and so don't leave a white mark), with the theoretical risk that they might enter the bloodstream. Concerns have been raised about the ability of titanium dioxide, once in the body, to affect DNA. The US National Institute for Occupational Safety and Health considers it a "potential occupational carcinogen".

Dr. Hauschka and Green People products also use light-deflecting ingredients.

Self-tan lotion

Green People has produced the world's first organic natural self-tan lotion without aluminium or other heavy metals.

Sunbeds and self-tanning

Some studies suggest that exposure to the UV rays used in sunbeds may cause the breakdown of folic acid in the body. In the first 12 weeks of pregnancy, when folic acid protects against spina bifida and other defects of the baby's neural tube, it would be sensible to avoid them.

Sun-avoidance strategies

Skin cancer experts and dermatologists now say sunscreens should be your third-line sun defence strategy after getting out of the sun and covering up well.

* Stay out of the sun between 11am and 4pm: even 10 minutes' exposure can burn fair skin.
* Wear a wide-brimmed hat or sunshades with a UV filter (the darker the better).
* Cover up in thin layers of natural fabrics.
* Drink enough water to keep your urine pale.
* Boost natural sources of betacarotene, lutein and zeaxanthin in your diet, which can protect against sun damage – make a tropical fruit salad from papaya, honeydew melon, nectarines, black grapes, kiwi, apricots and mango, or munch more carrots, spinach, red pepper, leeks and peas.
* Reset your expectations of summer skin by repeating the mantra "Tanned skin is prematurely aged and damaged skin".

Some pregnant women report nausea and headaches when using sunbeds, although there's no conclusive evidence to show that they are dangerous in pregnancy. But when your skin is extra-sensitive and subject to extreme hormonal changes do you really want to expose it to damaging UV radiation that worsens chloasma (see page 40) and greatly increases your risk of developing melanoma, a skin cancer able to spread to the placenta?

Sunbeds (if you can get on them) also can raise your body temperature dangerously high.

Self-tanning lotions might look like the best alternative, but, as with sunscreen, you risk applying a mix of chemicals widely over the body without rinsing off if you don't choose chemical-free formulations.

The best option in pregnancy might be to accept that pale is beautiful.

Remedies for skin problems

Try these safe homemade remedies to help alleviate some of the most common skin problems that pregnancy brings, including stretchmarks and dry, irritated skin. Many of them might help to de-stress mind and body – stress can aggravate skin problems such as eczema and psoriasis – and encourage you to rest more (the only sure remedy for undereye bags). These simple home cures might stop you reaching for off-the-shelf skincare products that could contain controversial ingredients, from formaldehyde to unsafe herbs.

Irritated skin

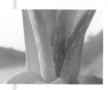 When it stretches tight and thins because of hormone changes, skin can become irritated and break out in rashes or even eczema. Avoid biological washing powders, and switch to "green" home products and DIY materials (see pages 56-59). If chlorine-treated swimming pools affect you, look for an ozone-treated alternative.

Beauty cure Liquidize half a cucumber and apply over the skin as a mask (avoiding the eyes – place refrigerated slices over them). Rest for 10-20 minutes before wiping away and splashing with cool water.

Bath cure To a tepid bath, add 6 drops essential oil of frankincense just before stepping in, swishing to disperse.

Dry, flaky skin

If your bed is flaky in the morning, it's time to take action.

Food cure Foods rich in essential fatty acids – nuts, seeds, small oily fish – are good for skin and baby. For vitamin A, eat red, yellow, orange and dark green fruit and veg, eggs, cheese and butter. Also eat foods containing vitamin B5 (meat, fish, wholegrains, pulses and nuts).

Massage cure Into 5 tsp apricot kernel oil and 1 tsp jojoba, blend 1 drop each essential oils of sandalwood (to moisturize), neroli (to rebalance sebum production) and patchouli (to heal cracked skin) and use for massage.

Beauty cure Place 1 bag lime blossom (tillieul) tea in a mug and pour over boiling water. Steep for 20 minutes, then soak a cotton ball and use to tone face and neck.

Perspiration

As your metabolism speeds up and blood circulates more rapidly during pregnancy, so you sweat more. Progesterone also dilates blood vessels and increases body temperature. Try these alternatives to talc and conventional anti-perspirants.

Hydro cure Plunge your feet into a bowl of cool water; if it's really hot, add a tray of ice. Sip a long, cool glass of water with slices of lemon or lime.

Clothing cure Wear layers of cotton you can discard during the day. At night, use cotton sheets and natural fibre bedding, and keep a window open, even in winter.

Herbal cure Try deodorants based on witch hazel, aloe vera, lemon or salt crystals. Substitute cornstarch for talcum powder (it feels fabulous on the skin).

Breakouts and acne

Pregnancy hormones are responsible for increasing (even overproducing) levels of sebum in the skin, which can cause pores to become blocked with shed cells, attracting bacteria and leading to inflammation. As you were 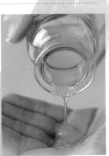 told as a teenager, cut back on fried, fatty, sugary foods and drink water to help flush out waste products the body now finds harder to process. Never squeeze or pick! Try to chill (see pages 68-69) – acne is worsened by stress.

Food cure Fill up on good sources of vitamin B3 – dairy products, oily fish and chicken, nuts, yeast extract and cereals.

Beauty cure Follow the cleansing routine recommended for your skin type on pages 24-25. Then soak a cotton ball in rosewater or orange blossom water and wipe the affected area. Dab on a little manuka honey, a potent antibacterial and renowned zit-zapper that acts on bacterial growth and soothes without drying the skin. Alternatively, substitute a little natural yogurt, beaten egg white (or clay mask for its drawing action) and leave to dry. Rinse off by splashing with cool water.

Massage cure Into 2 tbsp grapeseed oil, blend 1 drop each essential oils of bergaptene-free bergamot (for excess sebum), patchouli (to combat blackheads) and petitgrain (to close pores). Use a little to massage the face.

Herbal cure Smooth witch hazel gel over the affected area.

Thread veins

Tiny red veins or clusters of dots on the cheeks and shins may appear worse in pregnancy as blood vessels dilate and constrict more rapidly than usual, making them extra sensitive.

Beauty cure Make a toner from a vascular-constrictor herb: pour boiling water over 1 bag of camomile or marigold tea in a mug and steep for 5 minutes. Allow to cool, then soak a cotton ball for toning after cleansing.

Massage cure To 1 tsp peach kernel oil, add 1 drop each essential oils of neroli and sandalwood. Massage gently over the affected area.

Clothing cure Cover up in very hot, humid climes and in cold, windy places, too, to prevent the weather ravaging your face further.

Itchy skin

When skin is stretched tight across your belly, the urge to itch can disturb your sleep and may be debilitating. If, after 28 weeks, itching is very intense, 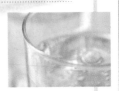 consult your healthcare provider. This may be obstetric cholestasis, a medical emergency.

Massage cure Soothe skin by rubbing in handfuls of organic olive oil after a bedtime bath while your skin is still damp.

Bath cure Take an easing oatmeal or rich oil bath, soothing irritated skin by rubbing with an oatmeal bag (see page 77). Alternatively, add 1 cup raspberry vinegar to the water.

Food cure Fill up on foods rich in vitamin B6 such as bananas, whole grains, peas and beans. Eat olive oil and drink plenty of water.

Remedies for skin problems

Chloasma

Ninety percent of pregnant women notice a change in skin pigmentation. Blotchy skin around the cheeks, forehead and neck that worsens in sunlight (becoming darker on pale skin, lighter on 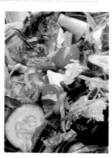 dark skin) is caused by the hormone that stimulates the melanocyte cells producing the pigment melanin. Melanin absorbs ultraviolet light and responds to the damage of UV radiation by tanning. The same hormone is responsible for darkened nipples and the line (linea nigra) down the centre of the tummy. Chloasma may fade eventually, but is very difficult to erase completely, even for dermatologists using high-tech bleaching agents and laser treatment. The best way to guard against it is to stay out of the sun and avoid sunbeds.

Clothing cure Cover up outdoors with a wide-brim dark cotton hat and huge, dark sunshades.

Food cure Lack of folic acid may worsen the condition: make sure you're taking the recommended daily supplement (400 micrograms) as well as boosting your diet with the ever-useful green leafy veg and other food sources of folate (oranges, chicken, nuts and seeds). Stock up also on foods containing PABA (para-aminobenzoic acid), found in wholegrains, fruit and vegetables including mushrooms.

Stretchmarks

Skin that expands rapidly across a swelling belly, breasts, upper thighs and buttocks equals stretchmarks for 90 percent of women (the scars of tears in connective tissue). Whether you get marks or not seems very much to do with genetics. Did your mother avoid them? Then you're likely to have inherited similarly elastic skin. The purplish brownness fades to silvery after pregnancy, but marks won't heal completely for years.

Food cure Increase your intake of zinc.

Massage cure To make a traditional massage oil for stretchmarks, mix 4 drops each essential oils of mandarin, neroli and frankincense, plus 2 drops bergamot in 2 tbsp sweet almond oil, 1 tsp wheatgerm oil and the contents of 1 vitamin E capsule. Use for gentle massage morning and night. (Avoid exposing skin to sunlight for 6 hours after use – citrus oils can cause phototoxicity. Omit wheatgerm oil if sensitive to wheat; substitute sunflower if allergic to nuts). Alternatively, massage with cocoa butter every day during the last two trimesters, or buy one of the many natural products available (see page 29). The founder of Belli cosmetics, Annette Rubin, recommends those containing the plant extract darutoside to speed healing and tissue regeneration.

Natural haircare

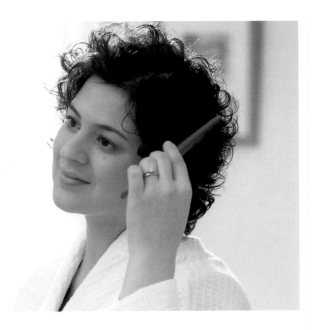

Oestrogen encourages hair growth and as you don't experience regular hair loss for nine months, your mane can appear lustrous, thicker and longer. (Make the most of it: hair is shed at an alarming rate after birth). One of the most common worries during pregnancy is whether it's safe to colour hair. This becomes more of an issue as we leave pregnancy till our thirties. Stress can be detrimental to hair health, too – a hunched neck and shoulders prevent good blood circulation and can add to bad hair days. The antidote – exercise and deep breathing, fresh air, good food, lots of water, a little massage and above all enough rest and relaxation is the best way to safeguard your health.

Everyday conditioning

For dry hair

After washing, massage into the ends of the hair 1 beaten egg mixed well with 1 tsp avocado oil. Rinse thoroughly with cool water.

For oily hair

After washing, massage into the hair 1 beaten egg, mixed well with 3 tbsp natural yogurt. Rinse thoroughly with cool water.

More intensive conditioning

Prewash for extra dry hair

2 tbsp coconut oil
2 tbsp runny honey
1 egg, beaten

Mix the ingredients together, whisking in the egg well, then massage into hair and scalp, combing through to the ends. Cover with a shower cap and

Natural high and lowlights

* **Dark hair** After shampooing, rinse with 1 cup strong black tea or an espresso (cooled) with a little vinegar and 2 drops essential oil of sandalwood, 1 drop rosewood. Or (wearing gloves) add a little walnut oil to a conditioning oil (see page 43).
* **Fair hair** After shampooing, rinse with a camomile/saffron infusion: place 1 camomile teabag and 1 pinch saffron strands in a mug, pour over boiling water and steep for 20 minutes; add the juice of half a lemon (try to avoid dousing the scalp itself).
* **Red highlights** After shampooing, rinse with a rosehip/clove infusion. Place 1 rosehip teabag in a mug with 1 tsp crushed cloves, pour over boiling water and steep for 20 minutes. Alternatively, make the final rinse with the cooled water from boiling peeled beetroot for 20 minutes (avoid if you have very light hair).

Japanese head massage

Bringing circulation to the hair follicles through massage is thought in Japan to be the secret of a naturally glossy head of hair. It is said to boost the uptake of nutrients in massage oils to aid healthy growth, making it the perfect safe beauty treat for pregnancy. It also relieves tension and de-stressing is always going to make you look better. It may also prevent dandruff, reducing the need for fungicidal shampoos.

If you can't get out of the house to the hair salon, try this home lock-lustre treatment. It works best on dry hair. If you don't mind washing your hair afterward, apply a little sunflower oil to your fingertips before you begin.

1 Start the blood circulating to the scalp by tapping lightly all over with your fingers. Bounce them over the scalp, then tap around the top of your opposite shoulder with a loose fist. Repeat on the other shoulder.

2 Place your thumbs at your temples, little fingers on your hairline at the centre of your forehead. Tense your fingers slightly, then make circular motions with each finger, rotating the skin over the underlying bone. Move back a little and repeat the rotations, working up and over the top of the skull and down to the nape of the neck.

3 Place your knuckles at the back of your neck. Ripple them around the nape of your neck and down toward the shoulders. Squeeze and release the tops of the shoulders between your fingers and palms. Pay attention to areas of tension, working carefully and feeling them ease.

4 Place your opened fingers, like rakes, into the hair at the crown of your head. Zig zag your fingers down through the hair on each side of the head, then repeat at the back of

your head, working all the way down.

5 Grasp handfuls of hair in your fists, again starting at the crown and working back and down. Twist the lock, then pull briskly to increase circulation to the hair follicles. Shake your hands to rid yourself of negative energy.

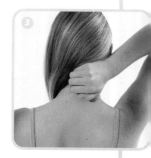

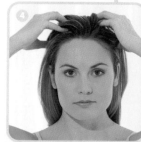

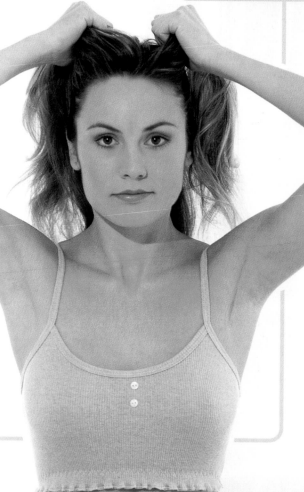

warmed towel while you relax for 30 minutes. Rinse away with cool water, then shampoo.

Prewash for oily hair

2 very ripe bananas

2 tbsp full-fat natural yogurt

Mash the bananas well and mix in the yogurt. Smear over your hair from the roots down, ensuring you work it through every inch. Cover with a shower cap, then a warmed towel and relax for 20 minutes or more. Rinse out with cool water, then shampoo.

Conditioning oils

Dry hair oil

3 tbsp coconut oil

1 tbsp avocado oil

6 drops essential oil of sandalwood or rosewood

Oily hair oil

3 tbsp peach kernel oil

1 tbsp jojoba

5 drops essential oil of bergamot (omit if using in the daytime)

Coloured hair oil

3 tbsp sweet almond or grapeseed oil

1 tbsp coconut oil

4 drops essential oil of ylang ylang

Damaged hair oil

3 tbsp macadamia or rosehip oil

1 tbsp avocado oil

4 drops essential oil of frankincense

Conditioning oil treatment

This twice-a-week treatment is especially effective on hair that has become dry, brittle or bushy. Work your chosen oil blend into dry hair; leave for at least 1 hour. When you come to shampoo off, work this, too, into dry, oily hair before wetting to help absorb excess oil.

1 Place an old towel over your shoulders and mix up an oil blend to suit your hair type from the recipes, left.

2 Pour a little of the oil blend into one palm and rub between both palms to warm. Place your palms flat over the sides of your head and make large, circular rotations, feeling the scalp move over the underlying bone. Move back a little and repeat, until you have covered every part of the scalp.

3 Apply a little more oil to your palms. Starting at the hairline above your face, take a section of hair and massage the oil blend into the length of the shank, making sure to cover from root to tip. Repeat up over the scalp to the nape of the neck.

4 Wrap your head in an old warmed towel and retire to bed, covering the pillow with another towel. In the morning, shampoo, condition and style as usual.

Natural colour washes

Talk to your hairdresser about using semi-permanent vegetable colours. At home try henna. Pure henna (do check the pack) is not, like many hair colourants, created from a long list of chemicals. Look for premixed varieties that cover every base from chestnut to blue-black. It does, however, have a distinctive scent that can make even the non-pregnant feel queasy. And once on, it doesn't come off again and can't be covered successfully – you'll have to wait for it to grow out or get a short cut if you hate the tone.

Off-the-shelf alternatives

Daniel Galvin Junior A high street product without SLF, sulphates, alcohol or phthalates that's rated even by hairdressers. Contains some organic ingredients. Daniel Galvin recommends Calming Baby Shampoo for pregnancy.

Aveda Multinational with eco credentials; phthalates have been banned since 2003.

Jurlique Sandalwood Shampoo and Sandalwood Herbal Protein Conditioner are formulated for hair damaged by styling and colouring and so suit brittle pregnancy hair and dry scalps.

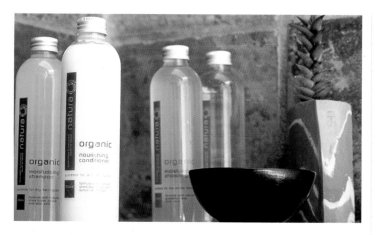

Weleda Calendula Shampoo and Conditioner are blended to suit those with sensitive scalps.
REN Try the Moringa Shampoo and Monoi Conditioner for dry conditions.
Living Nature Balancing and Revitalizing Shampoo and Manuka Nourishing Conditioner are based on soothing manuka honey scented with orange oil and contain jojoba oil, good for a scaly scalp.
Green People Vitamin Shampoo and Conditioner suit those who swim in chlorine-treated pools. Green alternatives to dandruff products, Itch Away Shampoo and Conditioner, contain bromelain extract from pineapple to rebalance a flaky scalp.
Try also: Paul Penders and Organic Blue; for Afro Hair try Burt's Bees Avocado Butter.

Non-toxic remedies for hair problems

Lacklustre hair

Food cure A diet rich in fruit and vegetables, fibre, protein and plenty of water only benefits your hair and health. Small oily fish and seaweed contribute vital oils and iodine, while olive oil, nuts and seeds bring on more omega-3 and -6 fatty acids and GLA (gamma-linoleic acid), thought to be metabolized into the hair to retain moisture and repair damage. Hairboosting vitamins and minerals are Bs and E, selenium, zinc and iron (eaten with vitamin C to aid absorption).
Herbal cure After the final water rinse, pour over plant-based cleansing rinses to restore the hair shaft's acid mantle. This increases shine. To remove built-up hair product, add half a cup of cider vinegar to the final rinse water. This also helps fight dandruff. To combat a dull, matte lifelessness, add nettle tea to the final rinse water (put 1 tea bag in a cup, pour over boiling water and allow to steep for 20 minutes).

Scaly scalp

Massage cure Mix together 1 tbsp finely ground sea salt, 1 tbsp runny honey and 1 tsp mustard oil. Massage handfuls into a dry scalp, feeling the skin move over the scalp. Shower away well, then shampoo and condition as usual.

Dandruff

Prewash cure Massage 1 cup apple juice into the hair from roots to tips before shampooing.
Massage cure Combine 3 tsp each jojoba and grapeseed oil and 1 tsp coconut oil. Blend in 4 drops essential oil of sandalwood. Massage the oils into the hair and scalp, then cover with a plastic showercap and a warm towel. Leave on for up to an hour. Shampoo and condition as usual.

Body hair

Many women find body hair fuzzes more quickly than ever, becoming darker and more widespread. Some salons are not keen to carry out waxing treatments on pregnant women because of unforeseen skin reactions due to extra sensitivity during pregnancy. Home kits, too, feature warnings against use during these months. Depilatory cream must contain no more than 5 percent thioglycolic acid. It's obviously not a good idea to apply bleach to the skin either.
Herbal cure Probably the most natural option is shaving (if you can reach). Apply a thin layer of aloe vera gel instead of shaving cream (may contain DEHA). Soothing for nicks and softening for the skin, it also means you don't have to apply chemical moisturizers afterward.

Clean, healthy teeth

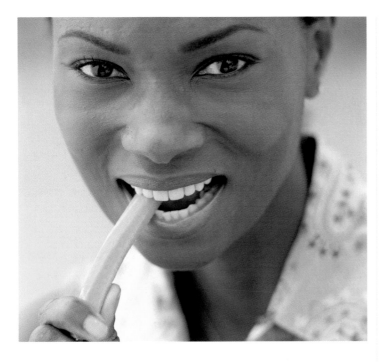

The health of your teeth during pregnancy links directly with the health of your baby, since pregnant women with serious gum disease run the risk of delivering early. It's important to visit the dentist during pregnancy (telling him about your condition and avoiding X-rays) to check out potential problems and get a good clean: built-up plaque is the most common cause of gum disease as well as tooth decay. If you're worried about using chemicals during pregnancy, toothpaste is a good place to start making changes, since mucous membranes in the mouth are remarkably permeable: over 90 percent of substances that touch them are swiftly absorbed into your bloodstream. Mercury amalgam fillings obviously aren't recommended during pregnancy: if you do need fillings have a good chat with your dentist about the alternatives.

Making natural cleansers

Salt cleansing paste In a dark glass container, mix equal quantities of fine sea salt and bicarbonate of soda. Replace the lid. To use, dip in a dry toothbrush, then brush.
Strawberries Rub over teeth and gums to remove stains and add sparkle.
Raw snacks At your desk, crunch on tooth-cleansing raw vegetable sticks, such as carrot, celery or red pepper, which also provide tooth-friendly vitamins.
Unwaxed organic lemons and oranges Rub the peel over teeth and gums to whiten and refresh.
Watercress and parsley Munch on these for a breath freshener, or boil up watercress and use the cooled water as a mouth rinse.

Making natural mouthwashes

Salt water Add 1 tsp antiseptic fine sea salt to 1 glass warm water and rinse well, especially if your gums bleed.
Green tea Place an (unflavoured) teabag in a cup, pour over boiling water, steep for 10 minutes and rinse the mouth – there's enough fluoride in green tea to reduce plaque and bacterial infections.
Nettle tea Place 1 bag in a mug, pour over boiling water and steep for 20 minutes. Use to rinse the mouth and spit out or swallow.
Lavender water and rose water Available on the cake-making aisle in the supermarket. Gargle and rinse, but don't swallow.

Off-the-shelf alternatives

If you're concerned, switch to a toothpaste that contains some or none of the above. Some "natural" toothpastes steer clear of peppermint and other substances that might interfere with homeopathic preparations. Read labels carefully; non-fluoride preparations may be formulated with ingredients you might like to avoid, while "natural" preparations might include fluoride.

For delicate gums

Weleda's Plant Gel Toothpaste is created to be gentle on delicate gums as well as tooth enamel. Green People Citrus Toothpaste treats sensitive gums with aloe vera to reduce swelling, immunity-boosting vitamin C and calcium carbonate for less abrasion.

Dentist approved

Kingfisher toothpastes, come with the approval of the British Dental Foundation.

"Natural" brands

Check ingredients listings to find something to suit you from Tom's of Maine, Nature's Gate, Logona and Desert Essence toothpastes.

Non-toxic remedies for gum problems

When you brush your teeth during pregnancy, increased blood volume in the area and the softening effects of progesterone cause gums to swell and bleeding is more common. Stress can aggravate this, and makes the mouth more acidic, a cause of tooth decay, so adopt also some of the de-stressing techniques on pages 64-93.

Tooth protection

Don't give up your cleansing regime when your gums bleed: plaque builds up more quickly in pregnancy and gums are more prone to infection. Try a softer toothbrush and be more gentle with floss.

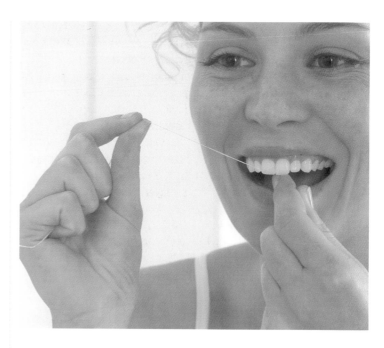

Brushing cure Use a tiny amount of toothpaste on a dry, soft brush, paying attention to where gums and teeth meet, circling gently round and round at back and front. Rinse very well. Keep flossing.

Food cure A diet high in the nutrients you need to protect your teeth has the benefit of helping your baby build bones, too. It also protects your bone density, guarding against osteoporosis in later life. Make sure you're getting enough magnesium and calcium (especially if you were excluding dairy from your diet before getting pregnant), protein, oils from small oily fish, and vitamins B, C and D

Bleeding Gums

Food cure Vitamin C-rich berries and citrus fruit, broccoli and potatoes strengthen capillary walls

and connective tissue, reducing the risk of bleeding. Eat a chunk of cheese after a meal to neutralize acids in the mouth that lead to tooth decay. Raisins contain bactera-suppressing chemicals.

Massage cure Massage gums night and morning with your fingertips, making small circular rotations all around.

Hydro cure If bleeding gums hurt, numb pain with an ice cube.

Breathing cure Breathe through your nose if possible to prevent saliva from drying out: saliva protects the gums and teeth.

Homeopathic cure Massage bleeding gums with a little of the homeopathic tincture hypercal.

Natural cosmetics

Health concerns may prompt you to "green" your cosmetics. Check ingredients listings where possible. The products recommended here are free from parabens, phthalates, and petrochemicals, as well as SLF, artificial colourings, flavourings and other questionable additives. Many are certified organic, and none are tested on animals. Best of all, every ingredient is listed on the label.

Bella Mama Products blended especially for pregnant women by a herbalist, aromatherapist and natural skincare specialist. Set up by two mothers in Colorado who found no existing products met their needs for natural, luxurious, organic skincare during pregnancy.
Belli Established by a former account executive at Estée Lauder, Annette Rubin, who was troubled by the safety of ingredients used in cosmetics for pregnant women. With her husband, a family practitioner, she developed a line using no harmful substances by correlating links between chemicals and birth defects.
Dr Hauschka German holistic products, including makeup. As natural as they come – not only are ingredients certified organic and grown biodynamically according to the cycles of the moon, they're also picked meditatively. Very good cleansers.
Earth Mama Angel Baby
Fab products and a super-informative website on everything from safe herbs for pregnancy to breastfeeding.

Erbaviva Californian organic and vegetarian products including anti-stretchmark brands.
Jurlique Biodynamically grown 98 percent organic products from a farm in a site of virtually nil pollution in South Australia. Branded as the "purest skincare on earth"! Try their day spa packages for pregnant women.
Living Nature Based on plants from the New Zealand bush, one of the "cleanest" places on earth, including manuka oil and honey, all suited to sensitive skin.
Neal's Yard Remedies Herbal-based products that include a certified organic range for mother and baby.
REN Set up when the founder's pregnant wife reacted to her regular skincare regime. Beautifully crafted quality products: the monoi body lotion for dry sensitive skin is so fragranced it's still discernible on skin the next day.
Selph High-end products for concerned pregnant women developed by the ex-Director of the skincare company Kiehls.
The Organic Pharmacy Very high quality products, favoured by stars such as Sarah Jessica Parker and Gwynneth Paltrow, created from organic oils by a pharmacist and homeopath.
Weleda Organic plant ingredients grown biodynamically and priced realistically from the famous Swiss-founded organization.
Try also: Organic Blue, Organica Botanica, Eveolution, Aesop, Beauty and the Bees, Doux Me, Anne

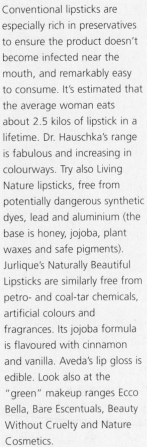

Psst... **Safe lipsticks**
Conventional lipsticks are especially rich in preservatives to ensure the product doesn't become infected near the mouth, and remarkably easy to consume. It's estimated that the average woman eats about 2.5 kilos of lipstick in a lifetime. Dr. Hauschka's range is fabulous and increasing in colourways. Try also Living Nature lipsticks, free from potentially dangerous synthetic dyes, lead and aluminium (the base is honey, jojoba, plant waxes and safe pigments). Jurlique's Naturally Beautiful Lipsticks are similarly free from petro- and coal-tar chemicals, artificial colours and fragrances. Its jojoba formula is flavoured with cinnamon and vanilla. Aveda's lip gloss is edible. Look also at the "green" makeup ranges Ecco Bella, Bare Escentuals, Beauty Without Cruelty and Nature Cosmetics.

Semonin, Just Pure, Lavera, Burt's Bees Baby Bees range, TerrEssentials, Aubrey, Avalon, Jason.

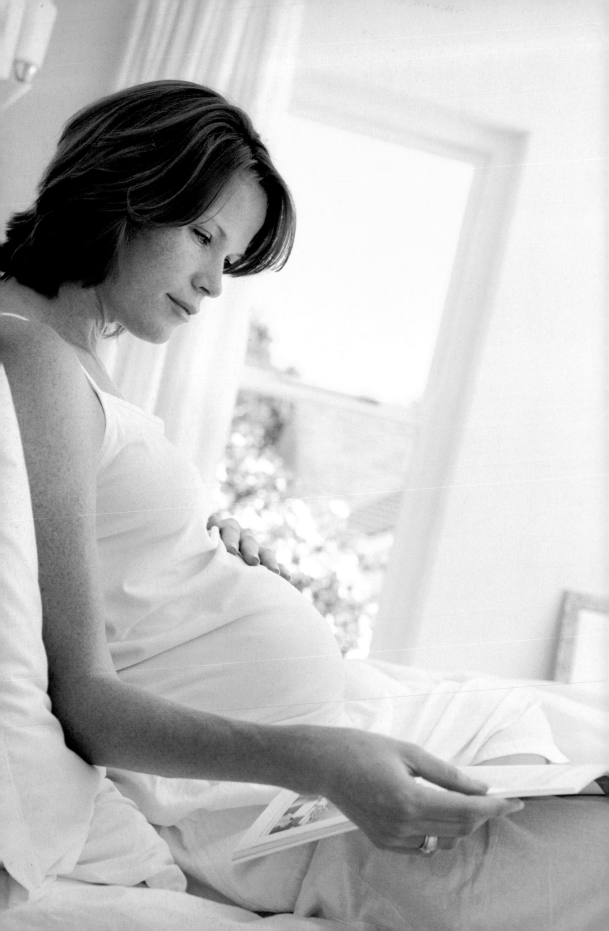

Your home sanctuary

You might think cutting back on commuting and less time spent in polluted city air would make your pregnancy healthier. But the average home contains more potentially dangerous chemicals than immediately outside its walls. Most are emitted from everyday products – mattresses to air fresheners, fabric softeners to TV screens – some of them three times more likely to be carcinogenic to humans than pollutants in dirty outdoor air. Open a window and breathe in some clean, nourishing air as you read how to make the rooms in your home less toxic.

"Greener" clothes

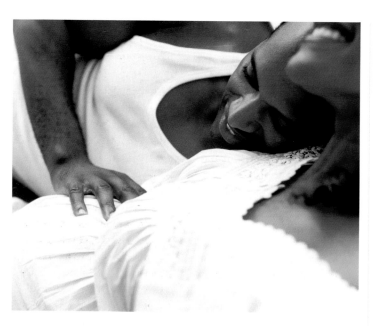

When you crave something natural against your skin to combat an itchy, sweaty pregnancy, you might opt for crisp white cotton. But the chemicals used to grow, bleach and treat this fabric could make it more toxic than some synthetic fibres. Organic cotton can appear whiter and waxier than regular cotton; companies selling it put this down to the health of the plants. Some claim it's softer to the touch, too, making it perfect for maternity underwear. Cotton raised organically may also be better in quality, since it can't be adulterated by mixing in mills with other grades of cotton. Hemp is a crop that thrives without pesticides and so is guaranteed residue-free; it can have a creamy texture quite unlike its scratchy image.

Organic products aren't cheap, but that's part of the ethos; companies like Patagonia and Howies urge you not to buy garments unless you really need and can afford them. In many new sustainable clothing companies, the garments are so well designed, produced and long-lasting, they'll become part of your life season after season: "consume less and consume better" they say. Howies' untreated selvage-edge jeans, for example, are made using twine 32 percent stronger and nine times more expensive than standard, woven slowly on a vintage shuttle loom in Japan. They improve with age. Slow Fashion takes inspiration from the slow food movement that promotes local produce and cooking methods over the instant gratification of global fast food.

Lingerie

Make toxin-free underwear and nightwear a priority: what's next to your skin all day and all night makes a difference. Wool and silk naturally wick away moisture, regulate body temperature and are antimicrobial. In organic cotton, try Blue Canoe's supportive sports bra for pregnancy; later their tank-style organic maternity bras without elastic or synthetic latex. Under the Nile has a nursing tank with inbuilt bra in organic cotton as well as nursing nightwear. German Sternlein cotton maternity tights meet some of the world's most stringent organic requirements. Greenfibres has an organic cotton maternity bra, plus a sports bra for pregnancy support and bustier for comfy sleeping – also check the luxurious undyed alpaca and Blue Face Leicester sheep bed socks. Schmidt Natural Clothing mail orders drop-cup or crossover-front nursing bras and nightdresses in organic cotton. For allergy/eczema sufferers, they recommend silk-cotton underwear; for everyone else wool and silk: the fabrics' biological structure resembles skin, making them very cocooning. Try the untreated, undyed socks and merino wool/silk vests and knickers.

Clothing care

Wool and silk don't need as much washing as plant fibre fabrics; their self-cleansing properties deter bacteria and fungi. Simple airing can even revitalize pure wool socks; hang outdoors overnight and allow dew to evaporate in the morning sun. Wash garments every now and then in cool water with an eco delicates liquid (no fabric conditioner) without rubbing or wringing which can break down fibres. Rinse in gallons of water; you could add ½ cup white vinegar to the final rinse for shine. Blot in a towel and suspend from a hanger to dry naturally or lie flat, never on a radiator. Be wary of tumble drying organic cotton garments: untreated fabric may shrink and need reshaping while damp.

Off-the-shelf "pure" alternatives

Blue Canoe (*www.bluecanoe.com*) sells Californian-Peruvian organic cotton in stylish styles and shades achieved with low-impact dyes. Pure, non-toxic underwear, tanks, pants and yogawear, plus soft bras for pregnancy sleeping.

Gossypium (*www.gossypium. co.uk*) offers fair-traded organic cotton clothes by working with the pioneering Indian eco organization Agrocel. Underwear and nightwear (expandable kaftan pyjamas), hoodies, t-shirts and yogawear are traceable from Gujarat field to hanger.

Greenfibres (*www.greenfibres. com*) sells ethically traded goods for home, body and baby from a company committed to UK-grown hemp. The underwear includes maternity staples.

H&M (*www.hm.com*) has phased PVC-brominated flame retardants,

phthalates, heavy metals, azo dyes, PCP and organotins from ranges without putting up prices or losing kudos (Karl Lagerfeld designed a range in 2004 and the maternity wear is a godsend).

Howies (*www.howies.co.uk*) are the best eco jeans and an award-winning base layer in 100 percent merino wool (a merino fleece is always better than its synthetic predecessor). Fab slogan t-shirts and organic cotton sweatwear.

Natural Collection (*www.naturalcollection.com*) is an emporium for hemp and other organic fibre underwear, socks and yoga clothes. Products and manufacturing processes are regulated by stringent guidelines to avoid materials known to be hazardous to the environment and health.

Marks and Spencer (*www.marks andspencer.com*) has one of the best eco policies, with organic cotton ranges developed with eco-conscious designer Katharine Hamnett.

Patagonia (*www.patagonia.com*) sells 100 percent organic cotton sportswear.

People Tree (*www.peopletree.co.uk*) is Tokyo /UK-based ecology fashion that supplies organic cotton uniforms for Aveda employees. Not only guaranteed free of chlorine bleach and unsafe dyes, these fair-traded clothes are created with crafts people around the world to revive traditional rural skills. Pieces get the Vogue vote for "modern urban

chic". The first fair trade organic line to be stocked by Selfridges. Also in store is Bono's wife's sexy ethical range, Edun.

Round Belly (*www.roundbelly. com*) offers everything in organic cotton for mothers-to-be, from maternity pants, dresses, work suits and party wear to underwear staples.

Schmidt Natural Clothing (*www.naturalclothing.co.uk*) are mail-order specialists in organic and untreated wool, cotton and silk. Especially fine underwear and nightwear.

Under the Nile (*www.underthenile.com*) supplies the best maternity shops with natural dyed, unbleached organic cotton garments with eco friendly fastenings. Good nursing pads and stylish nursing nightgown and bra.

Others to try: Eco Clothworks (*www.clothworks.co.uk*) and Ciel (*www.ciel.ltd.co.uk*); lust-after jeans from Dutch-based Kuyichi (*www.kuyichi.com*); glamorous hemp from Enamore (www.enamore.co.uk); and Kana Beach (*www.easyhemp.com*). Eco-ganik (www.ecoganik .com) fusing hip fashion with ecoconsciousness; Earth Creations (*www.earthcreations.net*) for clay-dyed hemp and yoga clothing; American Apparel (*www.american apparel.net*) for sweatshop-free tees and thongs in organic cotton; Rawganic (*www.rawganique.com*) for hemp everything from yoga clothes to sheets.

Low-tox bedding

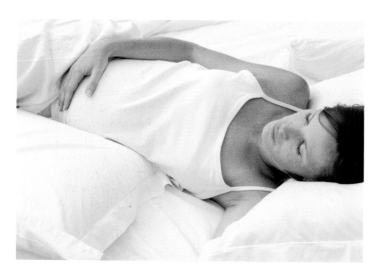

Mattresses

Look for untreated mattresses filled with naturally fire-retardant wool, natural rubber and latex, coir and horsehair that allow air to circulate. Real latex, like wool and coir, keeps you warm in winter and cool in summer, and has natural dust-mite and mildew resistance and antimicrobial action. Tapped from the *hevea brasiliensis* tree, natural latex is made up of millions of tiny bubbles that adapt to the contours of your body as they change through pregnancy, providing support and springiness where it's needed. Try a test run if allergic to the latex used to make gloves. In Europe, look for the QUL mark (the strictest German standard for latex mattresses). Natural mattresses might be covered in organic linen, cotton, untreated wool or hemp; the latter is becoming popular among mattress manufacturers for its immense durability – it's three times stronger than cotton. All can

be treated with the Indian botanical neem further to deter mites. To buy a non-wool mattress untreated with fire retardants in the US, you need a prescription from a doctor, chiropractor, naturopath or osteopath.

Mattress pads

If your budget won't stretch to a new mattress, choose thick woollen mattress pads from organically reared sheep or organic cotton wadding. Absorbent and insulating, they're a good buffer between you and mattress toxins. For waterproof covers, use wool "puddle pads".

Pillows

A lifesaver if you suffer pregnancy sleep complaints, try those filled with antiallergy buckwheat or millet. Both mould to your head, neck or bump as you shift in your sleep and still allow air to circulate. Contoured natural latex is a good alternative to memory foam

pillows, often chosen by people with fibromyalgia. Pure-grow wool pillows covered in organic cotton are the popular US eco choice, and are particularly good at wicking away moisture; we shed more from the scalp in sleep than any other body part. They don't plump down, and so maintain springiness. Mites, lice, mould and fungi also don't thrive in wool. If you can't sleep because you are uncomfortable, invest in a kapok body pillow – a bolster that matches the length of your body. Rest your top leg over when sleeping on your side.

Organic cotton sheets

Every organic supplier sells cotton sheets. Look for whites bleached with oxygen to avoid chlorine and optical whiteners, and colours achieved with "low-impact" dyes (or because the plant grows that way). Europe's best have the Dutch organic certification body's SKAL mark, the SWAN Scandinavian eco label, or Krav logo. Choose the highest thread count you can: 240-300 threads per inch means quality. Under the Nile has brushed cotton; Greenfibres stretchy cotton jersey and brushed cotton; Schmidt the crunchy crispness that comes from a 55 percent hemp mix; Rawganic 100 percent hemp fibres that that stand up to multiple washings. Dibb AB (*www.dibb.se*) sheets outperform the competition on napping, shrinkage, wear and tear, quality and eco points.

Duvets/comforters

Studies show wool is more comfortable than any other fibre to sleep under, keeping skin temperature and humidity at optimum levels for sleep comfort and lowered heart rate. Some companies sell light-as-air camel wool. If you love the soft merino wool blanket Scandinavian women buy to line their prams, get an adult-sized version for yourself. Schmidt organic wool blankets milled in Ireland double as a wrap.

Fleeces

Some mothers like to lie newborns in the daytime on a lamb fleece; many European mothers swear they keep babies comforted and temperature regulated at night, too, though midwives worry about overheating. If you don't want your newborn spending time on pesticide-dipped wool, look for organic fleeces that carry a certification mark, such as Yule fleeces from organic-raised Welsh lambs cured with substance derived from mimosa tree bark. Creamier in colour than chemically tanned fleeces, they are also noticeably softer, since no high temperatures are required in the tanning (extra oils remain in the wool, making it more naturally antiseptic).

Green bed brands

Alphabeds (*www.alphabeds.co.uk*). Small British manufacturer working with the Soil Association to establish a certification standard for mattresses based on the Dutch SKAL mark. Mattresses are free of flame-retardant chemicals yet carry the BS7177 safety label because they contain two or more layers of Welsh organic wool

Ecobedroom (*www.ecobedroom.com*). Every type of people-friendly beds and bedding from the Eco Living Center. .

Furnature (*www.furnature.com*) Non-toxic, odourless beds for the chemically sensitive.

Greenfibres For organically stuffed mattresses, raw untreated silk duvets and soft camelhair wares.

Hastens (*www.hastens.com*). Sleep like the Swedish royal family on a chemical-free mattress made the way they were in 1852.

Ikea For mattresses clear of known harmful fire retardants.

Natural Collection offers wool and latex mattresses, plus a good range of linens.

Natural Fibre Company (*www.thenaturalfibre.co.uk*). Undyed, unbleached Welsh blankets and throws from rare-breed sheep.

Nat Mat (*www.naturalmat.com*). The only chemical-free baby mattresses, bedding and linens to pass British safety standards: because your baby spends 60 percent of his first year asleep.

Organic Mattresses (*www.organicmattresses.com*) Just what it says.

Schmidt Natural Clothing supply wool mattresses and Demeter and Soil Association certified fleeces.

Psst... How do I care for eco bedding?

First thing, be slovenly. Don't make your bed on rising. Turn back the covers to let the mattress and underside of a quilt give up moisture. Then air quilts and blankets by throwing them out the window (think Middle European housewife). Once a month, hang bedding and pillows outdoors for a few hours in direct sunlight, if possible, to make the most of the natural bleaching and sanitizing UV rays. If it's raining, place in a drier on cool for 10-20 minutes with a tennis ball to fluff up fibres. To get rid of stains, mix 1 part white vinegar to 3 parts water, decant into a plant spray and spray the affected area. Allow to dry in sunlight. Wash cotton bedding and linen with eco powder (no softener). You can wash wool puddle pads in the machine on cold and line dry. Never dry clean eco bedding.

Shepherd's Dream (*www.shepherdsdream.com*). Wool bedding plus simple wooden beds and latex slats from the Californian pioneers of wool sleeping systems.

Green finishes & furnishings

Natural floor coverings

Wooden boards Reclaimed timber always looks good; seal with water-based varnish or eco floorpaint.

Linoleum All safe, natural ingredients. Linseed oil extracted from flax and pine tree resin bind fragments of cork, wood, clay and chalk to a jute backing. Not only low in flammability, lino is naturally antibacterial, sound insulating and oil-resistant.

Cork From the bark of a tree that is never cut down, this is the ultimate eco choice (when treated with a water-based sealant). Cork is naturally antimicrobial and insect-repellent, fire-retardant, wear-resistant and sound-dampening (it defies heels), warmth-regulating and cushioning. It doesn't outgas, nor shed particles that turn into dust. Cork is particularly good for bathrooms as it is impervious to water, does not rot and resists mould growth. It's totally degradable, not even giving off toxic gases when burned. Choose as tiles, roll-out sheets, or carpet underlay.

Bamboo flooring Robust and good in humid environments, bamboo grows without pesticides and is so tox-free that it can be composted after use if it hasn't been bound with formaldehyde-based glues.

Ceramic tiles, marble and slate Natural stone is a good non-toxic choice when you want a durable, hard surface for kitchens and bathrooms.

Cleaner carpets

Natural fibre If you can't live without wall-to-wall comfort, choose carpet made from wool, cotton or hemp. Wool is often the best option: naturally water-repellent, fire-retardant and air-trapping for good insulation, it's also more durable than most synthetics. Adding hemp to the mix brings extra mould, mildew and pest resistance plus durability.

Grass-based options From sustainable sources and often guaranteed free from pesticide residue, these woven fibres are hard-wearing and anti-static. Softest to the touch is jute, another naturally mould-resistant fabric (though moisture and sunlight cause it to break down). Durable seagrass is also quite comfortable, and has natural stain resistance. Sisal coverings are fire-resistant and good insulators, but rougher underfoot, and can soak up moisture, so don't suit bathrooms and kitchens. Coir comes from the husk of a coconut. This means it's itchily abrasive but also highly durable, and able to withstand exposure to water without rotting. It also repels insects, is naturally fire-retardant and a good insulator.

Natural backings Manufacturers are starting to introduce competitively priced alternatives to PVC-backing, perhaps because some big healthcare employers in North America are instigating PVC-avoidance policies. Look for untreated hemp and jute backings (they meet fire standards without PBDEs) bound with natural adhesive from the rubber plant.

Safer wall treatments

Eco glue/strippers Auro (*www.auro.co.uk*) sells a plant-resin DIY adhesive. Other companies have water-based, solvent-free paint strippers; OSMO (*www.osmouk.com*) sells a less toxic brush cleaner that thins oil paint.

Eco paints Less toxic (but more expensive) ingredients are low in VOCs and biocides (and biodegrade). They are marked "minimal/low-zero VOC", "VOC-free" or "no VOC". Be aware that adding colour adds VOCs. Some eco specialists offer "nursery-grade" options specially monitored to be extra non-tox. Ranges have expanded to include paints for bathroom and kitchen, floor, wood, metal, priming and outdoors. Ecos (*www.ecospaints.com*) offers an atmosphere-purifying paint based on silicate ingredients that absorb and neutralize airborne pollutants for five years. Try also Bioshield (*www.bioshieldpaint.com*) or Pristine Eco Spec (*www.texaspaint.com*).

Milk paints Manufactured using casein (a milk protein) and lime (calcium) with mineral pigments, most are extremely low in VOCs and naturally antifungal and antiseptic. Try Aglaia's washable distemper (*www.beeck.de*).

Linseed paint Solvent-free oil paints may be made from linseed or soya bean oil. They are nourishing for wood.

Water-based wood finishes Porous natural stains and seals based on seed oils, resins and beeswax allow wood to breathe and moisture evaporate, meaning they're less likely to crack or blister.

Eco papers At the top end come papers hand-printed with water-based acrylic or vegetable paints on fine or recycled paper. For uncoated versions, see *www.farrow-ball.com*. Then there are textured rice papers and plant fibre parchment: Try *www.phillipjeffries.com*, *www.shoptwenty2.com* and *www.innovationsusa.com*. Be sure to apply using a non-tox paste (make up with wheat flour, adding boric acid as an antimould insecticide). Some manufacturers create vinyl-look papers in sustainable natural materials such as cellulose. Others are experimenting with wall effects using jute, hemp, sisal and organic cotton, backed with fabric, natural latex or cellulose, perhaps toddlerproofed with a water-based sealant. You might also consider pressed wood veneers and woven woods, or even thin-split bamboo panels that roll out fine as paper.

Safer sofas

Seek out solid wood frames filled with natural rubber, wool, organic cotton and down, held together with water-based adhesives, finished with low-VOC sealants and stains, and upholstered in organic cotton. Then relax.

Sofa sources

Ikea: Lauded by Greenpeace for its furniture and furnishings.

Marks and Spencer: No longer uses penta- or octa-brominated fire retardants in sofas; it substitutes deca-brominated systems and has plans to replace all PBDEs:

US sources: Green building and furnishing store *www.greensage. com* offers sofas covered in organic cotton carrying the Swedish KRAV mark; *www.ecosofa.com* has a hemp-covered collection of organic sofas and easy chairs. Climatex upholstery fabrics (*www.climatex. com*) are 100 percent biodegradable. Also check the online organic lifestyle store *www.gaiam.com*.

Better blinds

Look for bamboo, fabric, metal and wooden slatted blinds, or Australian products; Australia leads the way in PVC-reduction programmes. EcoVeil blinds *www.mechoshade.com* are made from yarn. For more eco friendly building and decorating materials, check the US healthy building network site. *www.healthybuilding.net*.

Good wood

Sustainable hardwood is always the best option: instead of a changing table, try a regular hardwood table with hardwood shelves fixed to the wall. If you can't get away from composite woods, hardboard is

Psst... **Natural repellents**
Cedarwood blocks These are not a favourite fragrance of moths and fleas, so good for drawers and closets. You can even get cedar-filled pet beds.
Herbal deterrents Fill drawer sachets with dried lavender, white peppercorns, cloves, rosemary or mint. Natural Collection offers an earth-friendly repellent blended from cembra pine oil and carnauba wax.

least toxic, its wood chips bound with lignin (naturally occurring in wood). Or look for formaldehyde-free MDF (medium density fibreboard) compressed without adhesive. Ikea plywood products limit use of formaldehyde. Their solid wood children's furniture is treated only with water-based wax.

Cleaners

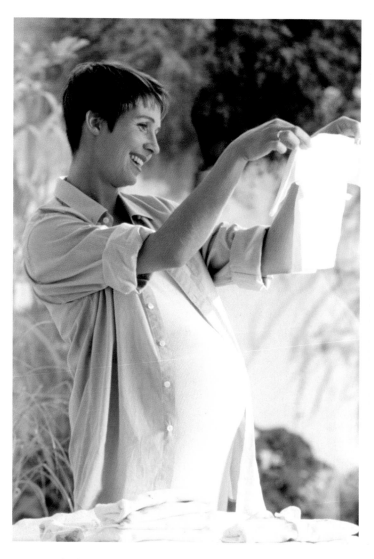

The synthetic fragrances we now associate with cleanliness are engineered to stick to clothing and bed linen and form a common source of skin irritation, especially when skin is super-sensitive. Aggressive artificial fragrancing can also irritate the nose and bring on pregnancy nausea. The good news is that modern eco laundry products perform as well as their dirty forebears, so you don't have to compromise on results as you protect your home (and our water sources) from environmentally alarming toxins.

Natural laundry products

Clothes/water softener Add $\frac{1}{2}$ cup white vinegar to the rinse cycle to reduce detergent residue in garments.

Static reducer Scrunch a ball of aluminium foil and pop in the dryer to reduce cling.

Stain remover Sponge on soda water (club soda), then wipe away; for more stubborn stains, apply a paste made by moistening bicarbonate of soda with soda water.

To cut through grease stains, mix equal parts white vinegar, borax and water; sponge on and wipe away.

White brightener Add $\frac{1}{2}$ cup lemon juice to the rinse cycle. Hang fabrics in the sun to dry.

Natural scent Dry laundry outdoors in sunlight. Fill the linen cupboard with bags of dried lavender or sweet-scented spices.

To rid new garments of chemical finishes Soak in a bucket of water containing 1 cup white vinegar.

Off-the-shelf alternatives

Although no laundry products are completely non-polluting, some are much less risky for your health and skin, the food chain and water sources. Look for those based on plant-derived materials that biodegrade rapidly and try using less (half at first, adjusting until you find the amount that suits your water type and washer).

Detergents

Ecover (see page 59) use non-GM protease and amylase enzymes that aren't active after washing. For the UK and German markets there's an enzyme-free washing powder. Phosphates are replaced with non-toxic polypeptides that break down in the environment. Tests ensure ingredients don't cling to fabrics after washing.

Seventh Generation (see page 59). For delicate pregnancy skin and babies try enzyme-free Sensitive Care Laundry Detergent formulated to clean without leaving irritating residue. For laundering first clothes, there's Natural Baby Liquid Laundry Detergent.

Bleach

Oxygen and hydrogen peroxide are much safer than chlorine. Ecover's Laundry Bleach is based on percarbonate, the next most natural bleach to sunshine, always the best bleaching option.

Stain removers

Schmidt Natural Clothing (www.naturalclothing.co.uk) mail orders an effective spot-removing bar based on gall for grease, paint and ink, blood and wine stains. Ecover's Stain Remover leaves no chemical residue.

Laundry balls

Laundry balls clean without powders or liquids and soften water naturally. Save water and energy because you don't need that second rinse (stops colours fading, too). Some people add eco bleach for whites.

Dryer balls reduce static and soften without chemicals or fragrances. Not that you'll be using your dryer if you care about the planet!

Psst... **Is your brand optically brightened?**

To check if your laundry powder contains synthetic brighteners, and to witness their longevity, coat your fingertip in powder and look at it under ultraviolet light. It will glow. Wash your hands and see how your finger keeps glowing.

Natural floor cleaning

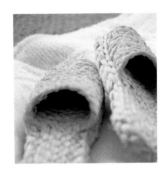

* Vacuum floors (plus upholstery and mattresses) using a cleaner fitted with a true-HEPA (High Efficiency Particulate Arresting) filter. It captures 95 percent of particles, unlike many vacuums that mobilize particulates back into circulating air to be redistributed around the home.
* Mop floors to trap toxic or lead-laced dust, rinsing well.
* Wipe over surfaces with a damp, lint-free cloth to immobilize dust (feather dusters and dry dusting just redistribute it). Or try sheep wool dusters, said to draw in dust with their electrostatic charge.
* Use a natural polish: Plain walnut oil; $\frac{1}{2}$ tsp olive oil blended with $\frac{1}{2}$ cup lemon juice; or 1 tsp white vinegar stirred into $\frac{1}{2}$ cup olive oil.
* Deodorize carpets by liberally shaking over bicarbonate of soda. Leave to settle overnight, then vacuum. Wash cotton, wool and other natural-fabric rugs twice a year to rid them of pesticides and toxin build-up.
* Once a year have carpets, rugs (and upholstery) professionally steam cleaned (check they're not using anything but water in the steaming device). In between, spot-clean stains using an eco friendly stain remover (see left).

Making natural cleaners

Kitchen surfaces
- Mix up half-and-half water and white vinegar in a pump spray. Spray over countertops, then wipe away (the vinegar scent disappears as the surface dries). To scrub off ingrained dirt, mix equal parts salt and vinegar and use with a scouring pad.

Stuck-on grime
- Fill a flour shaker with bicarbonate of soda (baking soda), sprinkle over and scour with a wire pad.

Ovens
- Prevent burnt-on grime by lining with aluminium foil to catch drips. Clean up spills while still warm and pliable. To remove burnt-on spills, mix bicarbonate of soda to a paste with water, apply over the oven interior, close the door and leave overnight. Next morning, scrub and wipe away, then wash out with liquid soap and water.

Chopping blocks
- Scrub with liquid soap and plenty of very hot water, rinsing well. For more abrasive cleaning and to remove stains, sprinkle with bicarbonate of soda, then scrub hard.

Disinfecting
- Add 8 drops essential oil of tea tree to 1 bucket water and use to wipe over surfaces or mop a floor. (Wear gloves.)

Dishwasher
- Sprinkle bicarbonate of soda over dirty dishes, then use half the amount of dishwashing tablets recommended.

Fridge
- Dilute 1 tbsp borax powder in 1L warm water and wipe around the fridge interior to remove stains and odours.

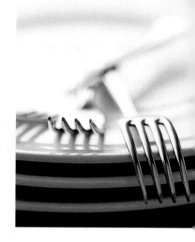

Drains
- Pour 2 kettles of boiling water down a drain. Pour 1 cup bicarbonate of soda down the drain, then 1 cup white vinegar. Cover and leave to fizz for 15 minutes, and flush with boiling water again. Use a drain strainer to stop food blockages.

Toilets
- Throw in 1 cup white vinegar and 2 tbsp bicarbonate of soda. Leave for 20 minutes, then scrub with a toilet brush before flushing. Alternatively, substitute the same amount of lemon juice and salt, or even baby powder and a can of Coke (a good way to wean yourself off both).

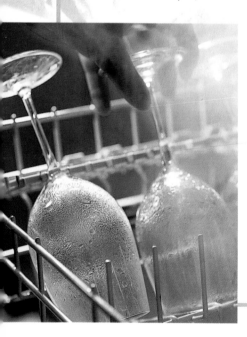

Baths and tiles

- Mix 2 parts borax powder with 12 parts white vinegar and lots of hot water. For less stubborn stains, simply blend equal parts white vinegar and water. Sponge or spray on, leave for 20 minutes, then wipe away. This should help clear mildew and mould.

Mould

- Wipe away as it forms using liquid soap and water, strong black tea or the bath mix above. After leaks and flooding, remove damp carpets, wallpaper and other items within 24 hours. Expose affected areas to sunlight or an ultraviolet (blue) lightbulb.

Wooden floors

- Pour 1 cup white vinegar into 1 bucket water and use to mop the floor to remove stains and smells.

Windows

- Mix equal parts white vinegar and water, then add 2 tbsp lemon juice. Decant into a spray bottle for use. Wipe away with newspaper.

Off-the-shelf alternatives

Ecover *www.ecover.com.* Europe's leading eco cleaning company reports that many women turn to its purer products for the first time in pregnancy. The washing-up liquid with camomile and milk whey, when tested for toxicity by organisms ultra-sensitive to water pollution, was found 40 times less toxic than the market-leading brand. Tests show products perform as well as conventional counterparts.

Seventh Generation *www.seventhgeneration.com.* With an ethos based on the Great Law of the Iroquois Confederacy, "In our every deliberation we must consider the impact of our decisions on the next seven generations", this is North America's most informative green cleaning company. Download a *NonToxic Home Guide* and subscribe to *Non-Toxic Times*. Petrochemical ingredients have been replaced with traditional favourites, such as vinegar, coconut and citrus oils and natural enzymes that perform like regular cleaners (and outperform other natural brands), but "won't turn your home into a toxic waste site". The Free & Clear products are for people who are dye- and fragrance-sensitive.

Microfibre cloths These cleaning cloths don't require cleaning fluids to remove stains; just dampen with water. Praised by many for their ability to rub away grease, dirt and dust like an eraser.

Safer pet products

Herbal deterrents Scatter dried lavender, white peppercorns, cloves, rosemary or mint around your pet's bed. Eucalyptus, citronella, sesame and neem oils also can deter fleas. Natural Collection offers an earth-friendly repellent blended from cembra pine oil and carnauba wax.

Instead of using insecticidal shampoos, treat your pet with your shampoo, leaving it on for more than five minutes to overpower fleas. Rinse well, then nit-comb. Launder pet bedding. Get a pet bed with a removable cover and wash weekly at a high temperature, especially during flea season.

Psst... **How do I get rid of dodgy cleaners?**

In your haste to get these toxins out of your home, don't pour bottles of bleach and disinfectant down the sink, toilet or drain, or chuck them in regular household waste. Call your refuse disposal people or Department of Public Works and ask about hazardous household waste collections. Or contact your local branch of Friends of the Earth or Greenpeace for advice.

Natural home fragrancing

Let fresh air in and toxins out

* Release airborne toxin build-up everyday by opening windows.
* Air bedding and soft covers outdoors occasionally.
* Let washing dry in the scent of blossom and roses outdoors. Do not expose it to fake scents in your tumble-dryer.
* Fit a fan in bathroom windows to permit air exchange and remove moisture.
* Sleep with a window open at night.

Perfume rooms with flowers and herbs

* In early spring, cultivate hyacinths or paper whites to drench a home with heavy perfume.
* In the summer, fill vases with cut roses, lilac and honeysuckle.
* Make winter pomanders: Puncture oranges with cloves and suspend from a ribbon.
* Plant up pots of scented herbs, such as lavender and rosemary, mint and lemon verbena. Brush them with your hand as you pass to release the fragrant oils.

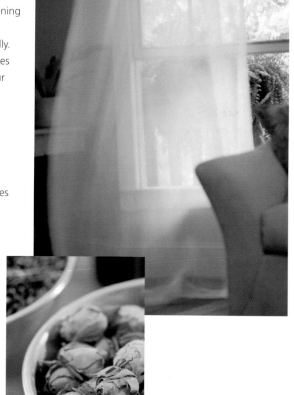

Use real scents and odour-eaters

* Choose artisan-made candles crafted from soybean oil or beeswax. Make sure they are naturally fragranced with real oils and botanicals, such as citrus zest and spices.
* Buy candles with cotton wicks for preference, or look for labels marked "lead-free".
* Add 8 drops of safe essential oils such as tea tree or grapefruit to the final rinse water when mopping the floor, or place 4 drops into the water bowl of a room vaporizer.
* Spritz flower waters around a room for a delicate mist of scent and to neutralize unpleasant odours, such as cigarette smoke and pet smells. Try Spiezia's Organic's Organic Baby Spritz.
* Leave a small bowl of bicarbonate of soda or white vinegar or half a lemon where kids can't reach it to absorb ugly kitchen odours.
* Dot a tiny amount of vanilla essence on a natural sponge and place in the fridge, kitchen or car.
* Bring a handful of cloves and broken cinnamon sticks to the boil in a little water, then simmer to scent a kitchen (watch that it doesn't boil dry).

Detox plants

Some houseplants actually crave toxins that can be dangerous in pregnancy: the leaves absorb chemicals that pass into the roots, where microbes turn them into food for the plant. Water pulled up from roots to leaves also sucks polluted air into the soil. The nearer the plants are to your nose, the more effective their purifying properties!

For your bedside table
- Christmas cactus (hybrid *Schlumbergera*): Unlike most plants, removes carbon dioxide at night and releases oxygen during the day, perfect while you're sleeping.
- *Dendrobium* orchid: Not just fabulously fashionable, it detoxes formaldehyde, acetone and chloroform from indoor air.

For the coffee table
- Areca palm (*Dypsis lutescens*): One of the best plants for removing airborne toxins.
- Lady palm (*Rhapis excelsa*): The second most effective detox plant, and are best for neutralizing ammonia from cleaning products.
- Bamboo palm (*Chamaedorea seifrizii*): Moisturizes centrally heated indoor air; good for removing trichloroethylene, benzene and formaldehyde.

By the computer
- Gerberas (*Gerbera jamesonii*): For instant cheer as well as effective toxin absorption.
- Golden pothos (*Epipremnum aureum*): Thrives in gloomy spaces with little natural light and loves formaldehyde.
- Dracaena (*Dracaena glauca*): A good detox plant that enjoys computer screen glare.

For the bathroom
- Boston fern (*Nephrolepis exalta*): The most effective air purifier, especially for formaldehyde; thrives in humid environments.
- Dwarf banana (*Musa acuminata*): Looks exotic and likes humidity.

For the kitchen
- Tulips: Grow bulbs indoors in early spring to remove xylene, formaldehyde and ammonia pumped into air by conventional cleaning products.
- Common peace lily (*Spathiphyllum "Mauna Loa"*): Siphons off VOCs (especially benzene) outgassed from flooring and wallpapers, paint and composite wood furniture, stain treatments and dry cleaned clothes.
- Spider plant (*Chlorophytum elatum*): Rids air of carbon monoxide and formaldehyde.

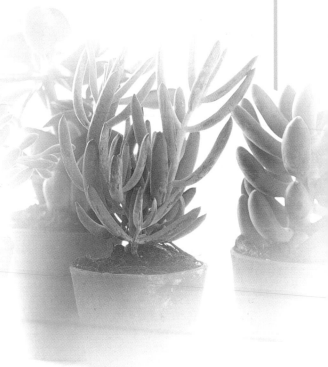

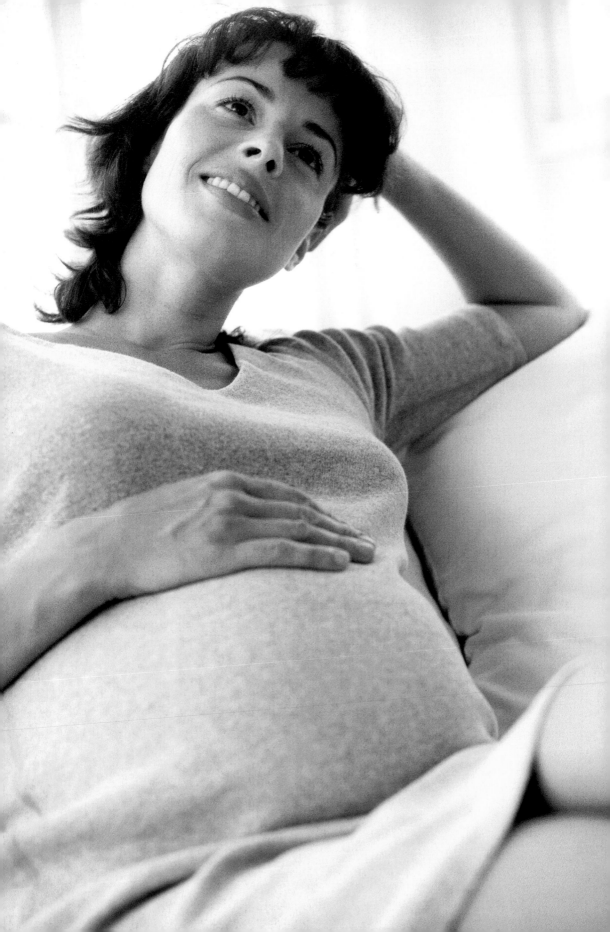

Easing stress

Pregnancy, especially for the first time, is fraught with self-doubt and fear. With each blood test and scan – if not every tuna sandwich and smoke-filled room – you find yourself awake at night pondering the negative possibilities. This is not good for your state of wellbeing, your baby or your relationship. Many of our own mothers say they enjoyed happier pregnancies than we do; they weren't expected to digest pregnancy manuals, scrutinize test results or worry about pesticides in food. Natural childbirth pioneer Michel Odent believes the months of pregnancy are too precious to be spent worrying; he urges mothers instead to "watch the moon and sing to their baby in the womb". Stress has been shown in many studies to be deleterious to the developing fetus and make low-level doses of chemicals in the home more damaging. This makes relaxing your body and resting your brain vital tools in your toxin-busting armoury.

The importance of relaxation

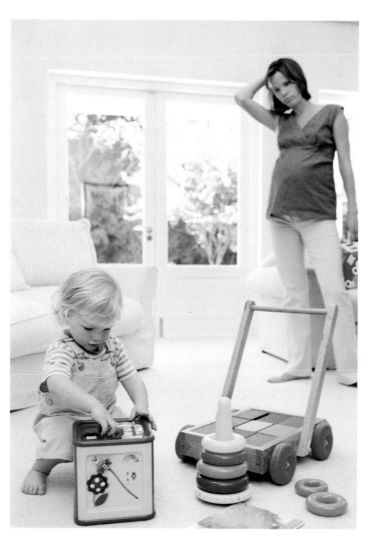

How stress builds

Worry brings with it physical change as the sympathetic autonomic nervous system primes the body to respond to stress by causing the release of a cocktail of chemicals, including adrenaline, into the bloodstream. As a result, heart rate, blood pressure, breathing and blood sugar levels increase. Blood, oxygen and energy flow away from the skin, digestive and immune systems toward the muscles and brain to equip them to react. The senses are also enhanced, hence the alert, racing thoughts and inability to focus that accompany times of stress. All these changes prepare us to overcome stressful situations by fleeing or fighting – the most effective ways humans have developed to deal with stressors such as predators. Reacting by punching or running kicks into action the parasympathetic branch of the nervous system to reverse symptoms such as a quickened heart rate. When we don't flee or fight, the physical build-up has no release, which can lead to anger, fatigue, raised susceptibility to infections and, over time, stress-related conditions from headaches to back pain. For pregnant women, living in a state of readiness to respond to stressors has been linked with changes in an unborn baby's brain development that may lead to physical and behavioural problems later in life.

Being worked off your feet, plagued by worry and guilt and wary about the changes taking place in your body and life only increases your toxic load. Many of us don't ease off work while pregnant. On the contrary. We rush to complete projects and set up foundations to keep things running smoothly in our absence, trying to cover every eventuality. On top of this comes the urge to make everything perfect for baby at home: at the least we scrub floors and repaint, and we may even knock down walls or move home. The result is stress in every area of life. How does this adversely affect your body and your growing baby?

When to rest

Whenever you feel tearful, tired, nauseous or ravenously hungry, see it as a sign to stop and take a walk, nap or snack. During the first and third trimesters, many women find they need a *siesta* after lunch and again on getting home from work. Lie down whenever the urge takes you without feeling guilty: you're only doing what's best for your baby. At your desk take regular breaks to stretch your limbs: this can stave off back and neck pain, swollen ankles and carpal tunnel syndrome in the wrists. When commuting, try to travel outside the rush hour and always demand a seat. Don't schedule every moment of your journey to be productive. Switch off and daydream: watch people passing, the changing cityscape, trees in bud or leaf and imagine your life in the very same season next year – with a baby.

Resting in the weeks before delivery

For your wellbeing and the health of your baby, you need to stop completely toward the end of pregnancy. For mothers in their late 30s and 40s this advice is particularly pertinent. By 32 weeks, try to give up work so you can rest whenever your body demands it. Women who have to work past 32 weeks are more likely to go into labour prematurely. By this stage, when all your organs are in overdrive and your spine and joints severely tested, you should not have to drag yourself out of bed early in the morning, and you deserve a daily *siesta* or two. Use enforced rest weeks to enjoy time with your family, partner and older children if you have them. Resting also reserves energy resources for the labour to come: if you are well rested and feel relaxed, you will find it easier to engage with the action and ride the waves of contractions.

How to unwind

It's not the stressor that matters; it's the way you react to it. Some people seem to cope well, even thrive, on stress; others get worn down by it. Luckily, it's easy to learn relaxation techniques that help neutralize the negative effects of stress: this chapter provides some effective methods.

Restful positions

Try some of these relaxing ways to de-stress at home and work. Forward-tilting positions not only relieve backache, they help ease your baby into the best position for labour – with the baby's back facing your front. In the last six weeks before the birth, try to adopt the following forward-leaning relaxation poses for 20 minutes twice a day or more.

Psst... Longterm effects?

A 2004 study showed that women who reported stress at 18 weeks of pregnancy were more likely to give birth to mixed handed children, linked with autism, dyslexia and hyperactivity. Other studies correlate stress in late pregnancy with behavioural and emotional problems in infants and in early pregnancy with preterm labour and low birthweight.

Watching TV

An adaptation of yoga's Child's Pose, this may be the only position that remains comfortable as your pregnancy progresses. Sit on your heels, knees open wide, and place pillows beneath your knees and feet and under your buttocks. Pile up large cushions, or a beanbag or birth ball, in front of you, then recline forward onto them, adjusting the support until you feel at ease.

Sitting at a desk or in the car

Sit on a cushion to raise your hips higher than your knees and make sure you take breaks frequently to walk around. In the office, if your chair is uncomfortable or makes your back ache, swap it for a regular dining chair and "customize" it until you find a

Progressive muscle relaxation

Appreciate the sensation of relaxation by contrasting it with tension. During the first trimester lie on your back – if it helps, cushion your head and the backs of your knees with a pillow and place another beneath your chest. After 16 weeks, lie on your left side or sit in a chair, feet on the floor.

1 If lying on your back, extend your legs away from you, feet wider than hip-width apart and dropping outward. Relax your arms away from your sides so that both shoulder blades are flat to the floor, and your palms are up and loosely open. If lying on your left side, bend your top leg forward and rest the knee and thigh on one or two pillows. Fold your upper arm comfortably. Close your eyes.

2 Start at the toes and feet: clench the muscles in the left foot tightly, lifting it a few inches; hold, then release. Feel the weight of your relaxed foot on the floor. Work upward, tightening and releasing your left calf and thigh, then repeat on the right leg. Feel the heaviness of your completely relaxed legs.

3 Tense your buttocks, gripping them and lifting slightly. Hold, then release. Pull your abdominal muscles in to cradle your baby and tense your chest. Let all the muscles in your torso relax, soften and spread.

4 Tense your left arm; clench the hand into a fist, then extend the fingers. Feel the arm shake with tension. Let the arm drop, totally relaxed. Repeat on the right arm. Tense your shoulders, pulling them tightly up and into the neck. Hold, then let everything go as you exhale and release.

5 Screw up your face, pursing your mouth, furrowing your forehead, screwing up your eyes and contracting your ears. Then yawn widely, opening your eyes, ears and mouth as wide as possible. Stick out your tongue. Release, letting go of the gripping in the jaw and forehead. Relax your tongue, ears, nostrils and the back of your scalp.

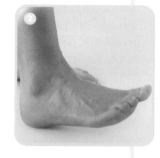

6 Scan your body from the toes up. When you find an area of tension, imagine it dissolving with the out-breath, and let the region melt into the support of the floor. Picture every part of your body soft and spreading outward and down, becoming heavier and warmer with each exhalation. Relax for up to 5 minutes. Stretch your limbs before getting up slowly, head last.

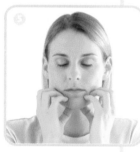

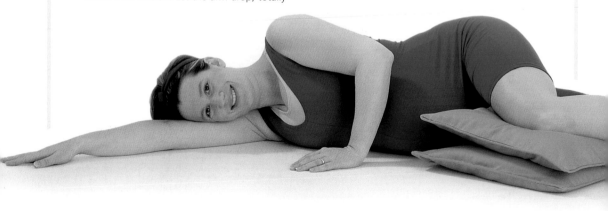

position in which you are comfortable. Turn it around, cushion the back and top, and lean forward onto it.

Easing aching legs
Elevate your feet when sitting to lessen the chance of developing varicose veins and swollen ankles. To make sure your lower back doesn't arch, place another cushion here to provide support.

Reading
Get into an all-fours position, hands beneath shoulders, knees beneath hips. Spread your fingers and flatten your palms to the floor, distributing your weight evenly between hands and knees and from right to left. Look down and place the book or magazine slightly forward to elongate your spine (don't let your lower back drop). Every few pages, rock your body forward and back, and circle your weight in one direction, then the other (a great position during birth to help the baby through the pelvis). When the weight gets too much for your wrists, sink back onto your hips, keeping your knees wide, and rest for a few minutes, arms stretching forward. This relieves back pain.

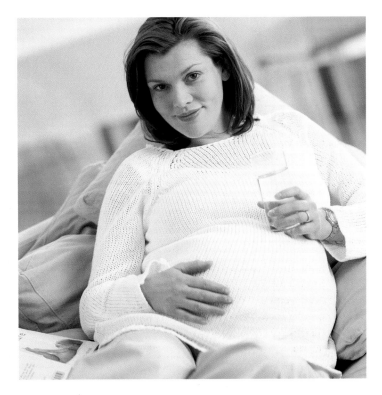

Relaxation pose

This restorative yoga pose relieves fatigue and stress-related headaches by boosting circulation to the upper body, which relaxes completely, supported by the floor. Taking the weight off your feet regenerates aching legs and helps prevent varicose veins and swollen ankles. Avoid after 16 weeks unless supervised by a pregnancy yoga teacher.

1 Sit with your buttocks and back pressing against a wall. Bend your knees and swivel to one side, buttocks still in contact with the wall. Then turn on to your back with both buttocks touching the wall and your spine flat to the ground. Take your legs one by one up the wall, knees slightly bent.

2 Relax your arms to the side, palms upward and open. Let your chest widen and relax. Release both shoulder blades to the floor, feeling them spreading out. Straighten your legs against the wall with each out-breath, pressing through the heels and both edges of the feet, as if supporting a weight on the soles. Hold for 30 seconds or more.

3 Open your legs wide until you feel a stretch through your inner thighs. Hold for 30 seconds, letting the stretch take your legs a little further down with each out-breath. Don't let the small of your back arch. Close your eyes or take your focus to your belly, watching it rise with the in-breath and fall with the exhalation. Reverse the movements you used to get into the pose to get out of it.

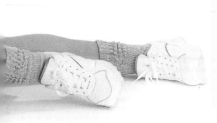

Relaxation breathing

Deep, controlled breathing is the essence of relaxation: it can reduce a raised heart rate and regulate blood pressure, help you let go of muscular tension and calm the mind by blocking stressful thoughts. More to the point, it can get you through labour drug-free. Use these techniques to maximize the flow of oxygen into your body and fully exhale stale air and waste products. This not only boosts the working of every part of your body (including the organs that eliminate toxins), it increases the amount of oxygen and nutrients available for your baby. If you can, practice outdoors in a relatively unpolluted place – by the seashore is good – filling your lungs with clean, fresh air.

Deepening the breath

Learn how to breathe more effectively, exhaling through a soft, open mouth unless this makes you feel nauseous. Each time you practice, change the cross of your legs to increase flexibility in the hips. In yoga this sitting position is thought to improve circulation in the legs and feet.

1 Sit on the floor with legs outstretched. Open your legs wide, then bend your knees, crossing your right shin comfortably over your left. Sit up straight, lifting out of your pelvis and feeling your sitting bones anchoring you to the floor. If you find it impossible to sit cross-legged with a straight spine, sit with buttocks, shoulders and head touching a wall. If this, too, is unbearable at first, sit on a firm chair with feet flat on the floor. As you practice over the weeks, work toward sitting unsupported on the floor. Close your eyes.

2 Place your hands low on your abdomen, one on each side of your baby. As you breathe in through your nose, bypass your chest and shoulders and imagine the breath dropping toward the abdomen, causing your fingertips to expand away from each other and the back of your waist and rib cage to expand, opening your chest.

3 As you exhale through soft, loose lips, picture the breath leaving your abdomen little by little from the top down and notice how your abdominal muscles draw toward your spine. This is one breath cycle. Take a regular breath, if necessary, then repeat the cycle for up to 3 minutes, noticing how your breath gradually lengthens and becomes deeper.

Counting the breath

Draw your mind away from outside disturbances by following your breathing. Counting the breath forces you to follow the action and stops stressful outside thoughts intruding.

1 Sit comfortably upright. Rest your hands on your thighs (relaxing your shoulders). Close your eyes and start to follow your regular breathing pattern.

2 When you feel at ease, breathe in to a count of four. Pause briefly, then breathe out to a count of four. Take a regular "recovery" breath, if necessary, then repeat the cycle for up to 3 minutes.

3 When you feel comfortable with the technique and no longer need to take recovery breaths, work on extending the out-breath: breathe in, as before, to the count of four, pause for four, then breathe out to a count of eight.

Using sound

An essential pain-relief technique that focuses attention on the out-breath. Don't worry if it feels embarrassing at first; practice where no one can hear.

1 Follow the deep breathing exercise on page 68, hands resting on thighs. When you feel at ease with the method, focus on the out-breath. Breathe in through your nose and sigh out through a soft, loose, open mouth, putting your voice behind it so an "Oooo" or "Ahhh" emerges. Don't worry about singing a pure tone, a groan is fine.

2 When the exhalation ends, close your lips and let the in-breath come naturally through your nose. Don't force or grasp at the breath. When you can breathe in no further, open your mouth loosely again and exhale with a noise, breathing out tension in the tummy, shoulders, pelvis, and, in particular, around your neck and jaw.

3 Repeat for 3-5 minutes, making the noise on the out-breath louder and less controlled, enjoying the relaxation this brings. Reach a crescendo, then gradually decrease the noise. After finishing, sit in silence with eyes closed for a few moments, feeling the intensity of the exercise.

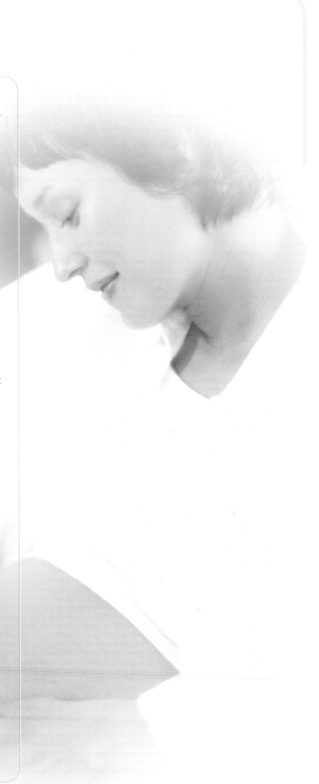

Relaxation breathing

Yoga Cat Pose

This moving breathing exercise gives every part of the spine a lovely stretch.

1 Start on hands and knees, legs hip-width apart with knees beneath hips and wrists beneath shoulders, fingers facing forward. Look down to align the spine from its base to the crown of your head, like a table top. Breathe in.

2 Exhaling, tuck your pelvis under, draw back your abdominal muscles, and press through your palms to arch your upper back toward the ceiling. Relax your head and neck. Hold briefly, waiting for the pause at the end of exhalation. As the in-breath comes, uncurl your pelvis and lengthen your coccyx away from the crown of your head, broadening your chest to form a table-top shape again.

3 When you reach the end of the in-breath, experience the pause, then, as you exhale, tuck your pelvis under to begin the upward arching again. Repeat the seamless undulation for 2 minutes.

Breathing with a partner

Teach this exercise to your birth partner. You won't use the leg movements during birth, but the linked breathing can be very comforting. In the labour room, you need support beyond words. When you are face-to-face with your partner, this comes in the form of his exhalation on your face reminding you to breathe.

1 Both of you should sit in Cobbler Pose (see page 88). Have your partner in kneel in front of you, placing his palms on your inner thighs.

2 Close your eyes and settle yourself by focusing on your breathing. Ask your partner to link his or her breathing with yours, mirroring your in- and out-breaths. After a few breath cycles, ask your partner to exert pressure on your thighs during the out-breath, pressing your knees toward the floor. Give feedback as to the amount of pressure you prefer, and ensure the pressure is lifted during the in-breath.

3 Work for 3-5 minutes, seeing how the out-breath lengthens as you work, and noting

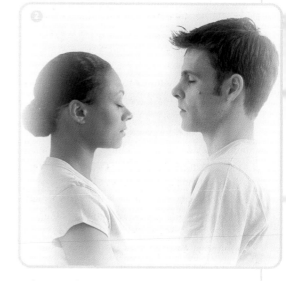

the natural pause at the end of the out-breath before the in-breath comes. This lovely stillness is accompanied by a little extra give in your legs, allowing them to descend a little further toward the floor.

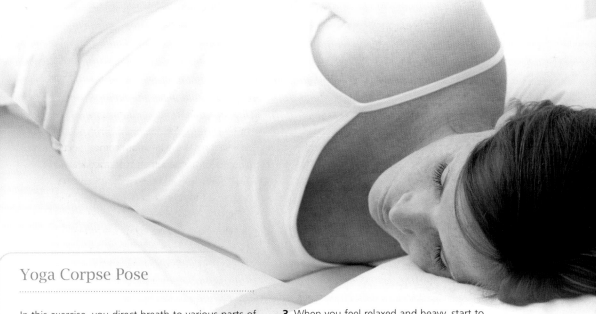

Yoga Corpse Pose

In this exercise, you direct breath to various parts of the body to release tension and energize your limbs. If you feel the cold, cover yourself from shoulders to toes with a soft blanket or shawl before you start. During the first trimester, lie on your back – if it helps, cushion your head and the backs of your knees with a pillow and place another beneath your chest to raise it. After 16 weeks, lie on your left side.

1 If lying on your back, extend your legs away from you, feet wider than hip-width apart and dropping outward. Relax your arms away from your sides so both shoulder blades are flat to the floor, palms up and loosely open. Lift your head only, look toward your toes to align it with your body, then replace on the floor, chin tucked in slightly to extend the back of the neck. If lying on your left side, bend your top leg forward and rest the knee and thigh on 1 or 2 pillows. Fold your upper arm comfortably. Close your eyes.

2 Use the muscle-relaxation technique (see page 66) to tense and relax every part of the body, starting at your toes and working up to your scalp. Then scan your body for residual tension and command it to release, allowing your body to sink into the firm support of the floor.

3 When you feel relaxed and heavy, start to focus on your breath. Watch your regular breath in and out for a while, then picture pulling the breath in through your toes and up your legs to nourish your baby with fresh oxygen and nutrients. As you breathe out, imagine pushing all your worries, physical tension and toxins out through your toes. Repeat a few times.

4 Next imagine pulling the breath in through your fingertips; as you inhale, pull the energy up your arms, around your shoulders and down your spine to nourish your baby. As you exhale, let your tension run out through your fingertips. Repeat a few times.

5 Finally, breathe in energy through your fingers and toes and let it run up your spine to the crown of your head. Imagine breathing out any remaining tension. Repeat a few times, then just relax, breathing regularly without letting your mind follow any thoughts. Relax for up to 20 minutes.

6 Wiggle your fingers and toes and stretch your limbs before coming to sitting. When you open your eyes, try to retain the sensation of energy and complete relaxation you felt during the exercise.

Meditation

With practice, meditation is the most effective way to empty the mind of preoccupations and restore a feeling of inner contentment often lacking at this time of change. Think of it as detoxing your mind. Meditation is effective when "pregnancy brain" prevents you from thinking clearly at work – it makes you feel more capable and alert, focused and efficient by optimizing brain functioning (it synchronizes brain waves between the left and right sides of the brain and boosts blood flow to the region). Meditation can be reassuring, too, when you can't sleep. That it is better at relaxing accumulated stress than sleep (or indeed any leisure activity) has been supported by many research studies. Meditation also offers a way to explore your changing body image and your developing relationship with your growing child.

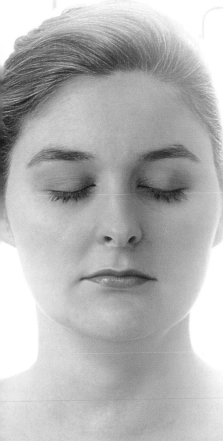

Clearing the mind

This is the most basic meditation technique. Use it to take time out and restore inner calm when you feel hyper-stressed, nervous or just plain angry: waiting for test results, reading about contaminants in our water supply or when no one will give up a seat on the bus. It can also ease nausea.

1 Try to sit with your spine upright, lower back supported, feet flat on the floor, palms resting on thighs. Whether sitting or standing, consciously relax your muscles, especially around the small of the back, neck and shoulders. Unclench your jaw, smooth out that frown and let your fingers and toes go loose. Breathing out, tilt your pelvis forward and up slightly to lengthen your lower back. As you exhale, feel your abdominal muscles engaging to cradle your baby. Broaden your chest (imagine opening a book, with your spine as the book's spine) to encourage deep breathing.

2 Close your eyes, if possible, and start to watch your regular breath moving in and out. Feel the in-breath cooling your nostrils; imagine the warmth of the out-breath contains all the body's toxins and tension. Let them go.

3 Watch your in-breaths deepen, expanding your abdomen and ribcage. Hear your exhalations lengthen. It may help you focus if you count the breaths, breathing in to a count of four and exhaling to a count of four.

4 Try to suspend the flow of thoughts through your brain by staying at one remove from them. Imagine your mind as a blank screen and see your thoughts as movies projected on the screen. Try not to follow the narrative of the thoughts (watching the movie). Wait patiently and the screen will go blank again.

5 Work in this way, observing your thoughts and disengaging from them, for 3-5 minutes at first, building up to 20 minutes' sitting practice with time.

Repeating mantras

Uttering a positive word or phrase over and over not only blocks out worry, it resets your default mechanism, making you sunnier in spirit. As you chant, your breathing becomes slower and more rhythmic, your mind fixes on the sound, and the repetition stills you. Medical studies show that chanting lowers blood pressure, slows the heart rate and boosts alpha brain waves to charge you with energy. Many people believe that sound waves can cleanse and revitalize body, mind and spirit.

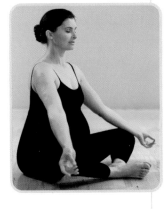

1 When you feel preoccupied or out of sorts, think of a word or phrase that makes you feel warm, calm and happy: perhaps "peace", "love", "relax", your baby's prospective name, or a reassuring phrase such as "everything will be all right". Roll the words around in your mind, uttering them quietly and pondering their significance. If one mantra doesn't hold your attention, try another.

2 When walking, let your chosen word echo to the rhythm of your footsteps. When painting or scrubbing the floor, feel it linking in with each sweep of the hand. Every time you repeat your mantra, feel its power lifting your state of mind.

Thinking yourself elsewhere

Guided imagery can ease you back into sleep during wakeful nights and may provide a place of refuge during labour.

1 Sit or lie comfortably and close your eyes. Follow your breathing, with each out-breath relaxing your muscles.

2 When you feel peaceful, think back to a time when you were completely happy and relaxed: lying on a beach bathed in warm sun perhaps; dozing with a sleeping baby warm on your chest; lying down after a fantastic meal; sitting in a secluded garden.

3 Take yourself back into the scene: hear the sounds, smell the scents, listen out for the sounds of nature. Immerse yourself so fully in this secret place that you escape from the world around you.

Psst... Just you and baby

At points in the day when there's a natural hiatus – on waking and before bed, at lunchtime and after work – stop what you're doing, quiet your body and mind, and look inside. Watch your breath move in and out for a few seconds and connect with your baby by "talking" to her. Visualize her body in its protective sac of fluid; imagine her lifeline, the umbilical cord, pulsating with energy. This need only take a few seconds, but keeps you in touch with what's important and stops stress from building. It can also help you say "no" to a tempting cigarette or additive-loaded snack.

Meditation

Nature walk

It sounds corny, but being pregnant makes you aware of nature: your own body seems to echo the changing seasons with their inevitable flow from sowing to growth and harvest. This fresh-air walking meditation helps you find this connection and has the power to shift worries and toxic thoughts.

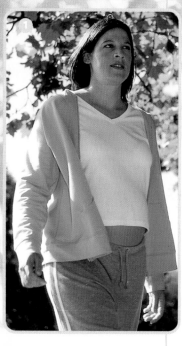

1 Go outdoors. Walk briskly for a few minutes to refresh your mind and senses. Take a few deep breaths and, along with the carbon dioxide, exhale your mental worries and physical aches and pains.

2 Let your breathing settle into the rhythm of your pace. Adjust your gait, doing a slight pelvic tilt and altering the length of your pace, if necessary, to support your lower back.

3 Start to notice the world around you. Look down at the earth and up at the sky. Feel the temperature of the air and search for clues to the season. Notice how your worries and physical tension seem less consuming.

4 Now slow your pace, making it more deliberate. Without looking at your feet, feel them lifting and being replaced on the ground. Be aware of your knees flexing and straightening. Notice how your weight transfers from your heel to the ball of your foot, then your toes. Note your new sense of balance as your centre of gravity has shifted through pregnancy.

5 Switch your focus to your breathing, inhaling for two paces and exhaling for two paces. When thoughts of where you're going or whence you came intrude, come back to awareness.

Using beads

For millennia, prayer beads have offered comfort to those going through change. The mechanical act of passing each bead through your fingertips draws you away from the world toward a tranquil place of stillness within. Try to find sandalwood or rose petal beads that give off a calming fragrance when rubbed.

1 Sit comfortably upright holding the beads in your right hand by your heart. Take the first regular bead after the large introductory bead or chain between your middle finger and thumb. Close your eyes and centre yourself by watching your breath, feeling it lengthen and deepen.

2 Inhale. As you exhale, roll the first bead between your middle finger and thumb, focusing on nothing but your breath and the bead.

3 Pass over each bead in the same way, linking the movement of your fingers with the rhythm of your lengthening in- and out-breaths. Each time your attention waivers, bring it back to the bead and the breath. Say a mantra on each bead, if you prefer (see page 73), or use words from your faith tradition.

Partner squat

An important part of de-stressing in pregnancy is learning to give up control and trust another force – in the squatting exercise below your birth partner; in real life, the force of contractions come all the more freely and less painfully if you go with them rather than tensing up.

Squatting is so effective because it broadens the pelvic outlet, easing the baby's journey down the twists and turns of the birth canal, and allows gravity to help push the baby out (maybe helping you achieve that desired drug-free delivery). This partner yoga also builds trust between you and your birthing partner.

1 Stand facing your partner. Place your feet hip-width apart, a few inches from your partner's feet and slightly turned out. Grasp arms by holding around each other's wrists. Stand tall, lifting your spine out of your pelvis. Breathing in, slowly raise onto tiptoes, mirroring each others' movements.

Hold briefly, then descend as slowly as you went up, this time breathing out. Repeat twice.

2 Both carefully lean back, until your arms are straight. Shift your weight so that neither partner is pulling the other off-balance. Relax backward without collapsing your chest and keep your pelvis lifting by tilting it forward and up slightly.

3 Exhaling, bend your knees and start to descend into a squat, as if sitting back on an imaginary chair, knees coming out in line with your feet. Inch down until your thighs make a right angle with the floor, then ease your buttocks down to your heels, attempting to get your heels flat on the floor. Try to hold here for up to 30 seconds, easily supporting each other and breathing evenly.

4 Inhale as you come up to standing together. Repeat 2 or 3 times. As you increase in confidence about your partner's support, lean back more: this makes the movement easier.

Cleansing candle meditations

An Indian meditation that calms and cleanses the mind by absorbing you in a physical focus of a flame. It's ideal when your thoughts are all over the place and you can't stop fidgeting, and works well in the bath (place the candle at the end by the taps). Beeswax is the least toxic choice of candle.

1 Sit comfortably upright on the floor, back supported if necessary, hands resting on thighs or knees. Place a candle on a low table, level with your eyes.

2 Settle yourself by watching your breath moving in and out for a moment, then focus on the tip of the flame, at the point at which its form and colour disappear.

3 Keep your gaze steady and uninterrupted on the flame for up to 60 seconds, trying not to blink. Then close your eyes and visualize the flame in your mind's eye. Let it cleanse your mind by burning away any intrusive thoughts.

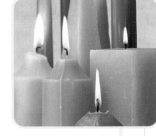

4 When the image fades, open your eyes and repeat the gaze. As thoughts intrude, just let them burn away and return to the flame. Work for 2-3 minutes.

Relaxation baths

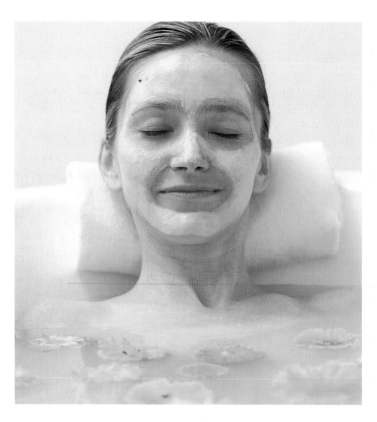

Nothing rejuvenates body and mood quite so effortlessly as a long, relaxing bath. In warm water, muscle tension ebbs away, the mind lets go and babies respond by turning somersaults of joy. Most commercial bath products contain substances that may be hormone-disrupting and many spa treatments are contraindicated during pregnancy, so here are some safe all-natural bath treats to ensure total relaxation. For peace of mind, select organic produce. If you are concerned about exposing yourself to toxins in tap water, be aware that toxins penetrate skin more efficiently when it has been softened by warm water and steamy bathrooms permit the inhalation of chemicals such as chlorine in water. Some pregnant women choose to fit a water filter to the tap or shower head.

Cautions: Do not take very hot baths during pregnancy; keep the water temperature tepid to warm, from a refreshing 75°F/24°C to a warming 95°F/35°C. Avoid saunas, steam rooms and whirlpool baths.

Ingredients to avoid

Pay particular attention to parfum, foaming agents such as SLF and PEG, PEG and artificial colourants. Soaking in warm water makes the skin 20 percent more able to absorb ingredients in bath products, making it especially important to avoid potential dangers.

Fizzy bath bombs

Some natural health experts recommend opening a window to reduce irritation from inhaling fragrancing ingredients.

Bubble baths

As they can be harmful to the health of the genito-urinary tract, these are best avoided if you are prone to urinary infections. Try an oil or milk bath instead (see right).

Non-toxic baths

To relax the mind

Flower bath Scatter a few handfuls of rose petals or lavender flowers over the bath water just before you step in.

Candlelit bath In the evening, turn off electric lights and fill your bathroom with beeswax candles. Close your eyes and inhale the scent of honey.

Vanilla bath Cast 4 vanilla pods into the water as you run the bath. Its scent has been shown in studies to lessen anxiety and induce relaxation. After the bath, dry the pods and reserve for another bath.

Sandalwood shower Into 2 tbsp unscented organic shower gel, drop 2 drops essential oil of sandalwood and 1 drop essential oil of patchouli, mixing well. Use to wash in the shower or pour under a running tap for a bubble bath. Sandalwood is an age-old recipe for peaceful meditation; patchouli helps to relieve anxiety.

Bedtime bath Just before stepping in, add 4 drops essential oil of lavender, a renowned sleep-inducing oil. Avoid during the first trimester, since the oil is an emmenagogue (a uterine stimulant that promotes menstrual flow).

To relieve aches and pains

Warming ginger bath Grate 5 cm (2 in) of fresh ginger root, tie up in a square of muslin and float in the bath as the water runs. Ginger has the power to ease aches and pains and reduce swelling while settling the digestion and combating nausea.

Soothing oil bath Just before stepping into the water, pour in 1 tbsp avocado oil, 1 tsp

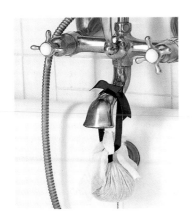

Baths for natural pain relief in labour

In the early stages of childbirth it can be comforting to climb into a deep, warm bath or birthing pool. Add nothing to the water, but if you're in for a while, top up the hot water to keep the temperature comfortable. Bathing is a good way to check whether this is real labour: if it's not your time, contractions will subside. When labour starts to hot up – contractions coming every 2–3 minutes and lasting up to a minute – stepping into a pool may help you stay in control and ride the waves of pain. Many women gain pain-relief during contractions by leaning forward over the side or end of the bath or pool. Between contractions, turn over or move around. From the leaning-forward position you can have someone mop your brow with a cooled wet washcloth or massage pressure points on your lower back for extra relief (see pages 82-83). Some women find being in water helps them squat, a vital position for assisting labour and relieving pain without drugs. Squatting becomes more comfortable when your body is supported by water, your back and arms resting against the side of a pool. The act of stepping out of warm water during labour can also be helpful – emerging into cool air can increase the urge to push.

wheatgerm oil and the contents of one vitamin E capsule (prick the capsule and squeeze in). Swish the oils well to disperse. This conditions very dry skin. (Omit wheatgerm oil if you are wheat-intolerant).

Milky oat bath Spoon 12 tbsp milk powder and 12 tbsp oatmeal into the centre of a large square of muslin. Tie to secure and cast into a bath as you run the water. Use the bath bag as an alternative to soap to cleanse the body; oats and milk are a proven antidote to itchy, irritated skin. (Avoid if you are allergic to milk).

To revive and renew

Cheering citrus bath To 1 tsp sunflower oil, add 3 drops each essential oils of orange and rosewood. Orange raises the spirits, and rosewood is a gentle, stress-lifting tonic. Avoid sunlight for six hours after use (citrus oils can cause phototoxicity).

Wake-up bath To 1 tsp grapeseed oil, add 4 drops essential oil of grapefruit, cleansing and stimulating when you need reviving after a hard day at work. Avoid sunlight for six hours after use (citrus oils can cause phototoxicity).

Top pregnancy herbs

Plants are powerful substances. Some may be toxic to the fetus, interfere with your hormonal or nervous system, or bring on contractions. It is always best to consult a herbalist or aromatherapist before use, but there ar remedies that can help alleviate stress and pregnancy ailments. Do keep your doctor informed of everything you self administer and make sure you buy your supplies from a reputable source.

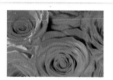

Lavender Placing 2 drops of essential oil on a pillow can help ease insomnia. Rubbing a drop of lavender on your temples can clear a headache. Rubbing 2 drops mixed with 2 tsp sweet almond oil over your abdomen can help reduce stretchmarks.

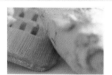

Ginger Sprinkle 1-3 drops essential oil of ginger on a tissue and inhale to help dispel morning sickness. Or drink ginger tea (see page 20) for the same result. It also may help with constipation.

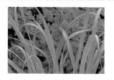

Rose Mix 1 drop of essential oil of rose with the contents of a vitamin E capsule and use to massage onto your perineum daily for one week before you due date to help soften the skin.

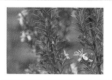

Lemongrass Place 4 drops essential oil in a water bowl of a room vaporizer to make a delightful air deodorizer. One drop added to another of peppermint to 4 tsp sunflower oil makes a good self-massage oil for heavy legs.

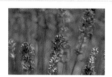

Rosemary This herb has a restorative effect on the nervous system. Sprinkle 3 drops of the essential oil on a tissue and inhale when you need to stay focused.

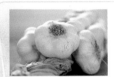

Garlic It will keep you well defended against bacterial and viral infection. It is also a powerful digestive stimulant, a mild laxative and can help regulate blood sugar. Add some to food as you cook.

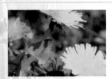

Dandelion The root and leaf are a traditional liver tonic, useful digestive stimulant and constipation easer. The leaves are high in iron; eat them in salads.

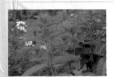

Peppermint Drink peppermint tea to relieve morning sickness as well as stomach discomfort. Place 1-3 drops of the essential oil on a tissue and inhale to fight nausea.

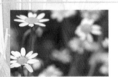

Camomile Try a cup of camomile tea to relieve morning sickness, particularly if you are feeling anxious or worried. This great relaxing drink also helps ease digestive disorders (see page 20).

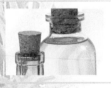

Tea tree Add 6 drops essential oil of tea tree to your bath daily for one week before a planned caesarian to help boost immunity.

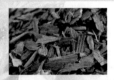

Rasberry Leaf Drink the tea in the last eight weeks to prime your uterus for labour. Also contains useful quantities of iron and calcium (see page 20).

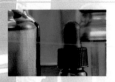

Rescue Remedy This combination of Bach Flower Essences is good for stress, tiredness and shock at any time, but comes into its own in labour. Take as directed between contractions.

Sleep promoters

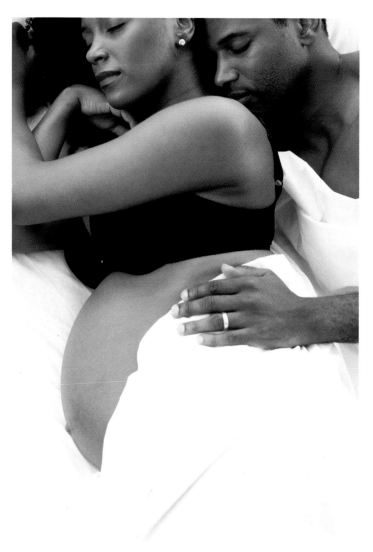

Psst... **Power napping**
When everything's getting on top of you and you can't think straight, it might be time for a daytime nap. A 20-60 minute power nap boosts brainpower, memory and alertness. But don't drift off for longer – this could make you drowsy and disturb your nighttime sleep.

The importance of sleep

Sleep is regenerative and, as it promotes the growth of cells, it is vital during pregnancy (not least for its ability to erase undereye bags). It boosts the immune system, which is lowered during pregnancy, helping fight off the negative effects of toxins, and promotes memory, so helping counter the forgetfulness that comes with late pregnancy. Above all, sleep is stress-relieving: during deep sleep the brain produces more alpha waves – those associated with quiet relaxation and receptivity – indicating that the body is relaxing and that the parasympathetic system (the nervous system that reverses the fight-or-flight stress response) is taking over.

Sleep positions

When it's impossible to sleep on your front, and dangerous to sleep on your back (weight can restrict

When you're exhausted, emotional and unsteady on your feet, all you crave is a good night's sleep. Certainly, this is the only beauty treatment guaranteed to restore fresh-looking skin and shining eyes: during sleep, the body secretes growth hormones that regenerate skin and hair. But when you hit the sack during pregnancy, inevitably you can't settle for an itching belly, restless legs and an inability to get comfortable. And when you finally drift off, it's only to be woken 20 minutes' later by an urgent urge to urinate. If this describes your regular pregnancy night, some natural remedies can be helpful.

the circulation of blood and oxygen through the major vein that supplies your baby), copious pillows are the answer. Lie on your left side to boost the flow of blood and nutrients to your baby. Bend your top leg forward, placing a pillow or two beneath your knee and thigh to support the knee and hip joints. This position also boosts kidney function. Tuck another pillow between your legs to support your lower back. Alternatively, search the web for pregnancy "wedge" pillows, specially moulded to fit the body.

Tips for getting back to sleep

- Get comfortable by rearranging your pillows.
- Banish a snoring partner to another room.
- Fit blackout blinds beneath curtains to keep the room dark.
- Try progressive muscle relaxation (see page 66) to ease aches and pains.
- Use a meditation technique (see pages 72-75) to switch off a racing brain.
- Focus on your breathing: breathe in through your nose for a count of four and out for a count of eight.
- If all else fails, get up and make yourself a milky drink, listen to some soporific music and read a dull book.

Deep sleep routine

1 Take regular aerobic exercise during the day as this promotes good sleep but avoid exercising within three hours of bedtime.

2 Make your bedroom inviting. Banish work, computers and other equipment that reminds you of tasks that must be done to another room. Keep the lighting soft with side lamps rather than glaring overhead bulbs. Open windows to get a good flow of fresh oxygen and rid your bedroom of stale air and bad vibes. Change bedding regularly; clean linen pressed with lavender water is comforting. Gather enough pillows to make yourself comfortable.

3 Have an early supper, leaving at least two or three hours before bed: eating late can lead to digestive problems that interrupt sleep. Don't drink caffeine in the evening (nor the afternoon if you suffer from insomnia badly).

4 An hour or so before bed, have a milky drink and something to eat containing l-tryptophan, an amino acid that encourages sleep. You'll find it in bananas, lettuce, wholemeal bread, crackers, turkey meat and eggs.

5 Write down everything you need to remember for the next day, then forget about it.

6 Wallow in a relaxing bath (see pages 76-77). Get dressed in clean nightwear and put on a sleep or soft sports bra to support your breasts, if necessary. Follow a bath with a relaxing massage (see pages 82-83) to ease residual muscle tension. Having someone rub your feet with oils when you can't reach them can be very sleep-inducing.

7 Meditate before getting into, or indeed once you're in bed (see pages 72-75). Meditation empties the mind of intrusive thoughts.

8 Read if it helps you relax, but keep it unexciting: thrilling page-turners are way too stimulating.

9 If you have the energy, lovemaking can be nicely soporific.

Massage

At any stage of life, massage is one of the most luxurious of stress-busting treats. Traditional Chinese Medicine recommends two massages a week during the last trimester to relieve tension, ease lower-back pain and swelling, and energize mind and body. Find a therapist who specializes in massage for pregnancy (and has a massage table with a cut-away section to accommodate your bump, or a heated water pad for back massage). By boosting circulation, massage helps the natural reduction of built-up metabolites (waste products), from tissue. It also boosts immune function. Some acupressure massage techniques are very effective at easing pain during labour, when being touched is also a reassuring reminder that you are loved. Make sure you teach them to your birth partner.

Self-massage strokes can be very helpful in relieving tension: Try the sequences for face, head, hands and feet on pages 27, 42, 31, 35.

Massaging the back

Enjoy this soporific sequence after work or before bed to relieve strained muscles and soothe nervous tension. Make it last at least 20 minutes to ensure the release of endorphins, the body's natural painkillers.

1 Sit on your heels, knees open wide, relaxing forward onto pillows (cushion also your feet, heels and knees, if desired). Have your partner kneel behind you.

2 With a little oil on his hands, your partner should place his palms on your lower back, one on each side of the spine, fingers pointing upward. He should stroke firmly up from lower back to shoulders, out over the tops of the shoulders and firmly down the sides of the body, drawing in at the back of the waist to return to the starting position. Repeat in a rhythmic flow for 3–5 minutes.

3 Place palms at the top of the shoulders, one on each side of the neck, and squeeze, releasing over the shoulders and down the upper arms. Repeat several times, paying particular attention to areas of tension. This can diffuse tension during labour, too.

4 Place knuckles on the shoulder blades and ripple them in a circular motion all around the area. Then exert pressure around the lower back (as in steps 2 and 3, opposite). Stroke down around the thighs and calves to the feet, rippling over the soles with the knuckles.

5 Finally, place both palms at the top of the shoulders, one on each side of the spine, and draw alternate palms in turn down the back; let the second hand begin the stroke as the first reaches the sacrum, building up a continual flow of strokes. Finish by resting palms on the lower back.

Massage for labour

Have your birth partner practise these strokes on you before everything kicks off: you probably won't feel like giving orders once labour is well-established. You do not need oil for these firm pressure techniques.

On lower back

1 Relax forward, chest well supported with cushions or against the back of a chair or bed headboard. Have your birth partner place his or her palms on your shoulders, and press downward to relax tension, then stroke firmly down either side of the spine with flat palms, building up a flow of strokes.

2 Have him position his palms on your pelvis on either side of the spine and exert firm pressure with the heels of his hands, hold, move an inch outward and repeat, working toward the hips.

3 Repeat using the thumbs, pressing quite firmly into the back of the pelvis using bodyweight, holding for a few seconds before circling, releasing and gliding an inch or so toward the hips to repeat. Repeat at the centre of each buttock outward.

On legs from standing

1 Stand facing a wall, an arm's distance away, feet hip-width apart. Take one pace forward with one foot and bend the front knee. Lean your upper body into the wall, feeling a stretch down your back calf.

2 Have your partner kneel by your back leg and firmly stroke down from thigh to calf. Some active birth teachers ask him to urge "Come on, baby" (at which point he should anticipate a kick). If it feels good, have him knead knotted muscles in the calf, too. Change legs and repeat.

Oils for massage

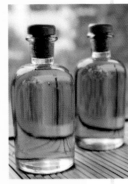

Oil helps the hands slide comfortably over the body and is great for conditioning dry skin. As the skin absorbs what's applied to it, this is also a good way to supply your body and baby with useful nutrients, including brain-friendly fats and essential vitamins and minerals. Go for the pure organic vegetable and nut oils recommended on pages 28-29. Some essential oils can be very helpful during pregnancy. Always mix them in a base or "carrier" oil, such as organic sunflower or olive oil, adding no more than 2 drops essential oil to every 2 tsp carrier oil. The following essential oils are particularly appropriate during pregnancy

* Rosewood for gently refreshing and easing nervous tension and tiredness.
* Citrus oils – grapefruit, mandarin, petitgrain and neroli – to lift the spirits.
* Ginger to ease nausea.
* Sandalwood to relieve anxiety and as a skin tonic.
* Ylang ylang to lift the spirits and banish feelings of panic.

Massage

Oils for pain relief

Pain causes heart rate and blood pressure to rise, and stimulates the release of the stress hormone cortisol. Some essential oils, including lavender and, to a lesser degree, rosemary, seem to have a stress-reducing effect, even if they do not change physiological responses to pain nor decrease pain sensation. In a 2004 study, people who inhaled essential oil of lavender while experiencing physical pain reported less awareness of the discomfort when recalling it later and seemed to suffer less anxiety during the experience. In labour only, try these:

* Lavender to reduce anxiety, stress and awareness of pain and to speed delivery. Add 2 drops essential oil to hot or cold water. Soak a washcloth in the water, wring out and apply to the lower back or forehead.
* Jasmine to strengthen contractions, relieve pain and lift the spirits. Add 4 drops essential oil to the water in the reservoir of a vaporizer.
* Neroli to ease shock and distress. Add 2 drops to a bowl of hot water and inhale if candle-powered vaporizers aren't allowed in the delivery room.
* Geranium to counter anxiety and balance the emotions. Use in a massage blend or compress.
* Rose to promote contractions and relieve nervous tension. Mix up a massage blend, adding no more than 2 drops essential oil to 2 tsp carrier oil.
* Frankincense to calm and deepen breathing. Add 1-2 drops essential oil to a handkerchief and sniff as required.
* Clary sage to speed contractions during a slow labour (only to be used by an aromatherapist).

Pelvic tilts

The most effective way to guard against damage to the pelvic floor muscles in pregnancy is to do pelvic squeezes everyday for the rest of your life. Remind yourself to do them each time you look at your watch or have a drink. Exercising and relaxing the muscles also helps them stretch efficiently during the second stage of labour and heal effectively after the birth. Start with pelvic tilts to bring your awareness to the region, then practice the lifts (see opposite).

1 Lie on your back until 16 weeks, when you should do pelvic tilts on all fours, hands beneath your shoulders, knees beneath your hips, spine perfectly flat, like a tabletop.
2 Breathing out, draw your abdominal muscles toward your lower spine and engage your buttock muscles to tilt your pelvis forward slightly. Feel your lower back arch (if lying on your back, there should be no gap between your lower back and the floor). Hold until the end of the out-breath.
3 Inhaling, release, feeling the muscles soften, and return to your starting position. Repeat for 1–2 minutes.

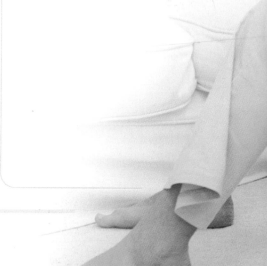

Perineal massage

In the last six weeks of pregnancy, natural birth gurus recommend a daily five-minute massage of the perineum, with oil to increase its elasticity and aid the intense stretching that comes with childbirth. This reduces the risk of tearing or the need for an episiotomy.

1 After a warm bath, when your skin is nicely supple, apply a little wheatgerm or olive oil to your fingers (avoid wheatgerm if you are wheat-intolerant).
2 Insert your thumb and index finger about 5 cm (2 in) into your vagina and gently press down toward your rectum and sideways. Hold until you feel a tingling sensation, like when you stretch your mouth open widely. Hold for 1–2 minutes until the burning subsides into numbness, then release.
3 Massage the inner part of the vagina for a few minutes.

Psst...leak prevention

In a 2004 University of Montreal study, 70 percent of women who regularly used exercise to strengthen the pelvic floor were cured of post-pregnancy incontinence within 8 weeks.

Pelvic floor lifts

1 Squeeze and lift the muscles around your vagina, as if trying to stop yourself urinating. Hold for 10 seconds (don't forget to breathe, keeping your stomach, legs and buttocks soft). Release, then push the muscles outward slightly. Repeat 10 times.
2 Squeeze as before; hold, then lift further; hold; lift a little more; hold for 10 seconds. Relax in stages.
3 Pull in the muscles around your anus. Hold for 10 seconds, then release. Repeat 10 times.
4 Squeeze as before, hold, then lift further and hold, lift a little more, and hold for 10 seconds before relaxing in stages.
5 Draw up all the muscles, contract them and squeeze quickly 10 times. Repeat 10 times.
6 Finally, squeeze and lift all the muscles, hold for 10 seconds, then squeeze and release them quickly 10 times. Repeat the steps whenever you remember, aiming for numerous repetitions a day.

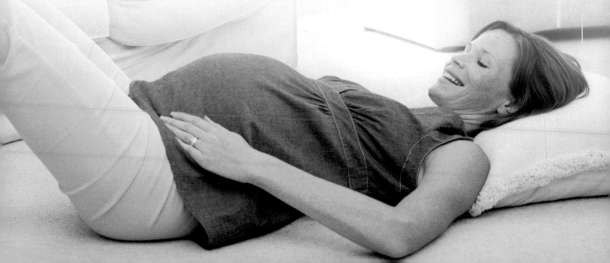

Stress-busting exercise

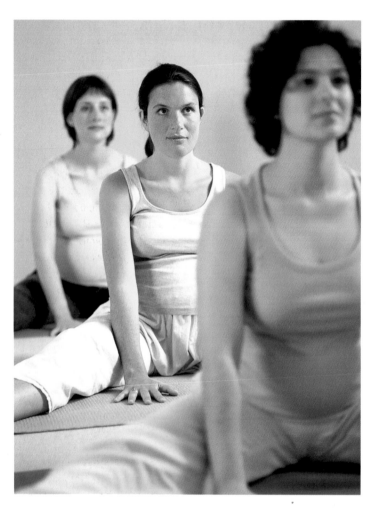

Good exercise choices

Yoga

The exercise *par excellence* from weeks 1 to 40 plus. Yoga poses focus your awareness on and strengthen the spine to enhance your posture and prevent backache. They also help restore balance, which shifts as you gain weight, preventing accidents and injury. Stretches expand the pelvic area and strengthen the legs to assist labour, and the breath control techniques may just get you through the birth drug-free. Some poses are said to encourage the release of stored toxins. Opt for a specialist antenatal class, and avoid "hot" or "power" yoga.

Pilates

Low-impact movements gently and precisely hone core muscles supporting the spine and pelvis. Breathing is linked with each movement and attention focused on how your abdominal muscles function, both helpful in labour. Attend an antenatal class with a teacher who has studied modified moves for pregnancy.

Exercise in water

Whether you choose a midwife-led class for pregnant women or just go swimming, be reassured that exercising in water is one of the best options in pregnancy. Water aids buoyancy, supporting that cumbersome body and vulnerable spine and joints, its temperature reduces the risk of overheating, and

Nothing helps combat stress and promote relaxation more effectively than exercise. Exercising is another good tool in your fight against toxins, since getting mobile also gets fat supplies mobile; converting fat into fuel releases fat-soluble chemicals to be sweated out of the body. It also boosts immunity. Research shows that women who exercise have less stressful pregnancies and seem to cope better with labour, requiring less medical intervention and pain-relief, and producing brainier babies. They also get back into shape more quickly after the birth.

Caution: Consult your doctor before beginning an exercise programme, especially if you have a medical condition, back or joint problems, or a history of miscarriage. Make sure you tell exercise instructors about your pregnancy.

the movements and holding of breath enable deep breathing. Water resistance gives a safe but potent cardiovascular and muscle-defining workout. Like yoga, it is safe to continue until the day of the birth. Seek out ozone or UV-treated pools, which require less chlorine.

Dancing

Line dancing, salsa and other types of dance that leave you mildly breathless and elated make perfect pregnancy exercise. Always bend the knees slightly and maintain a pelvic tilt to protect the lower back, and avoid twisting movements and sudden changes of direction. Belly dancing was developed by women in the Middle East for delivery. It frees the pelvic region, lengthens the spine, and yokes breath and emotion to the movements. The squatting action is great for strengthening leg muscles, too.

Walking

Easy, free and available to all, walking is many pregnant women's exercise of choice. Pregnancy professionals rate it for exercising the heart and lungs and toning the lower body in a low-impact way (it doesn't put unnecessary strain on unstable knees and ankles). If you're new to walking, build up slowly, resting every other day. Eventually, aim for 3 to 5 weekly sessions of 30 minutes or longer. Start and finish each workout at an easy pace, and in the middle of the session, take it up a level by

alternating your regular pace with 1–2 minute intervals of power walking (at a fast pace with arms pumping). As you get larger, stick to flat terrain and watch not to arch your lower back. Don't run or jog after the first trimester; it's uncomfortable for breasts and belly, and jarring for pliable joints.

Cycling

Just the kind of supported cardiovascular workout pregnant gym fiends crave. The cycling position also helps widen the pelvic outlet. Speed training is not the idea; keep the pace gentle.

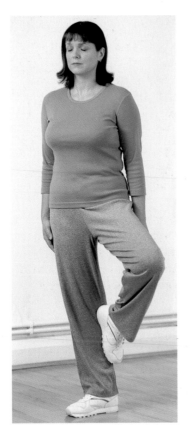

Classes for pregnancy

Low-impact aerobic or step classes for pregnant women with a trainer qualified to guide you safely through cardio, toning and stretching routines.

Sports to avoid

Contact or extreme sports, and those that might cause falls or strikes to the abdomen. This rules out skating, riding, downhill skiing and surfing; football, basketball and hockey; vigorous racket sports, gymnastics and kickboxing. Scuba diving is unsafe and you should also avoid exercising at altitudes above 6,000 feet.

Psst... Keep it safe
Beware overheating, which can reduce blood (and oxygen) flow to the fetus. Lack of hydration can bring on cramping and contractions. Inddors, stay near air vents and fans; outdoors avoid the hottest times of day for working out. Drink ½L (1 pint) water a couple of hours before exercise, then a glass every 15 minutes during a workout, in small sips.

Yoga for pregnancy

A pregnant woman's ideal yoga posture, Cobbler Pose helps open the pelvis and promotes bloodflow to the region. It boosts good posture by broadening the chest, and engages the abdominal muscles to support the lower back. King Pigeon Pose promotes circulation to the pelvis and opens the hips. Being a forward bend, it is also very relaxing. Active birth teachers consider the squat the most important pose of all for a healthy pregnancy and mobile labour. Follow these by relaxing in Corpse Pose (see page 71).

Cobbler Pose

1 Sit up straight with legs stretched out in front. If you can't sit upright without slouching, sit with your buttocks and back touching a wall. Spread your legs wide. Bend at the knees to bring your feet toward your groin, placing the heels and balls of the feet together. If your knees are very stiff, place cushions beneath each one.

2 Interlink your fingers and firmly grasp your toes (if this is too difficult, hold your ankles). Inhaling, stretch your spine up and feel an equal stretch through both sides of the body. As you exhale, draw your abdominal muscles back to support your lower back and tuck your chin in slightly to lengthen the back of your neck.

3 Without losing this feeling of lift, press your feet together and, exhaling, press your knees toward the floor. As you breathe in, broaden and lift your chest, roll your shoulders back and away from your ears.

4 Try to hold for up to three minutes. With each in-breath, grow taller, lengthening your waist and puffing out the chest. With each exhalation, let your knees drop a little lower, feel your abdominal muscles cradling your baby, and sense your pelvis anchoring you to the floor.

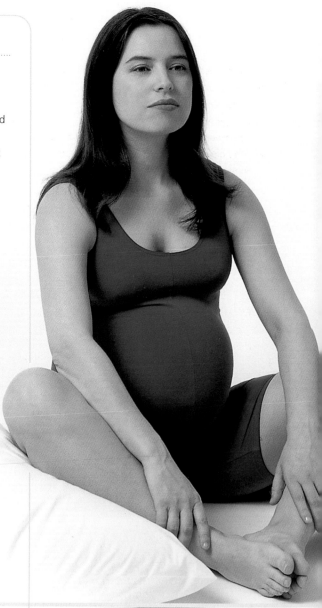

King Pigeon Pose

1 Sit up straight with legs stretched out in front. Place your palms on the floor beside your hips and press down to grow tall, pushing through your heels to straighten your legs and expanding your chest as you inhale. Hold for a few breath cycles, trying not to collapse in the lower back.

2 Move your hands forward slightly and manoeuvre your legs so the left leg is straight behind you, the right crossed in front of your bump at a right angle, foot flexed, heel aligned with your knee.

3 Breathing out, take your weight onto your hands and lean forward, keeping your spine straight from sitting bones to the crown of the head. Straighten your back leg and level your hips, feeling the stretch through your left front thigh and right outer hip. Pause here for a few breath cycles. Breathe out any discomfort.

4 When you feel ready, breathe in. Exhaling, lower your body further without rounding your back. Come to rest over your front leg supported on your elbows or, eventually, with arms outstretched in front. Breathe out tension in the hips and back thigh. Try to hold for 1 minute or more. Come up slowly on an inhalation, head last. Repeat on the other side.

Yoga Squat

1 Place your feet wider than hip-width apart, toes pointing outward. Breathing out, squat down, placing your palms on the floor in front of you for support, and drop your pelvis down.

2 When your buttocks reach your calves and your feet are flat on the floor, bring your elbows inside your inner thighs, place your palms together in prayer position, thumbs touching your sacrum, and press your elbows outward to widen the knees. Lengthen your spine, extending through the back of the neck, push your chest forward and drop your sitting bones. Hold for up to 3 minutes, breathing out discomfort with each out-breath.

Caution: Avoid overstretching; the hormone relaxin, which helps the uterus expand, also relaxes your connective tissue, making you impressively stretchy, but destabilizing the joints, inviting injury. After 16 weeks, avoid lying on your back and inversions. As your centre of gravity changes, hold a wall or bar during balance stretches if necessary.

Coping with change

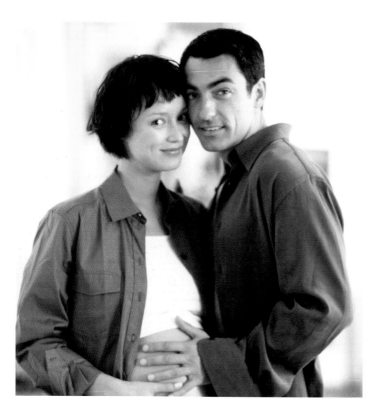

Pregnancy means confronting change, from the unstoppable swelling of your belly to the move from a work-centred life to a more home-focused universe. This can be disconcertingly stressful if you've been leading an "adult" life for decades, going out to do what you want, when you want and with whom you want. Intense change can make little things overwhelming, inconsequential worries stack up to bring on panic attacks in the middle of the night. When change gets you down, or you find yourself battling against it, counter anxiety with relaxation techniques and try some of these coping strategies to put you in a more confident and contented frame of mind.

Practical ways to dissolve worries

Financial issues

Find out about your entitlement to maternity and paternity benefit. Work out what you need to live on while away from work and what your income will be. Total up your debts, then try to work out a repayment plan (you might visit a financial advisor). It can be quite cheap to live with a baby: you go out less and so save on transport and entertainment costs. Review your list of "must-have" baby items; you actually don't need that much. Borrow as much as possible and investigate the range of secondhand baby shops.

Health concerns

Assuage doubts by getting informed about pregnancy and birth. Join active birth classes to learn how the pregnant body works; schedule extra appointments with your midwife or doctor if you think it will be helpful and won't worry you more; find out if your maternity unit has a 24-hour helpline; visit the place where you plan to give birth with your partner.

Relationship matters

Worrying about how a baby will change a relationship, and how a partner will cope is a source of stress for many women, especially older mothers-to-be with long-established lifestyles. Talk to your partner about your concerns, but be aware that it's almost impossible to imagine the reality of life with a baby however many books you read. Many couples find birth brings welcome release from worry about a nebulous future and empowers them just to be, working through issues as they arise.

Worries about toxins

Reassure yourself that you are doing all you can to rid your daily life of unnecessary chemicals by detoxing your home, makeup bag and food cupboards. Vote with your purse by buying organic food, eco home and green beauty products, then try to stop worrying.

Sharing fears

Talk it out

It can be difficult to admit to fears about pregnancy when everyone's telling you how good you look and how well you are coping. It can be especially hard to talk to a partner when fears about your relationship are dragging you down. Meeting women in the same situation might be the answer. Join a local antenatal yoga group for the exercise and also for socializing. You'll find everyone shares similar fears and you will build a network of shoulders to cry on after the birth, when life gets more crazy.

Have a cry

Almost everyone has times when it's all too much. Having a good cry on the shoulder of your partner, sister, mum or best friend can bring relief.

Simple treats

* Put your feet up and read a book or magazine.
* Go for a swim.
* After work, refuse to do anything until you've spent at least 30 minutes lounging in the bath.
* Take a taxi occasionally to escape the stress of a crowded bus.
* Buy a new outfit that makes you feel good about your new shape.
* Plan a holiday before the baby comes (check with airlines and your doctor).
* Have a pedicure every couple of weeks.
* Book a massage with a therapist who specializes in pregnancy.
* Take weekend breaks with your partner, indulging in lie-ins, afternoon lovemaking, bracing country walk, and unforgettable dinners.

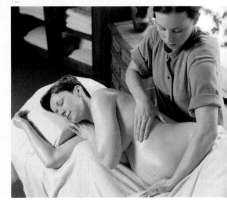

Nourish yourself

Eat well

Foods rich in B vitamins boost levels of the hormone serotonin, which has stress-busting properties.

Try flower remedies

Aspen deals with fear of the unknown. Agrimony might assist those who suffer in silence. White Chestnut can be helpful when the same concerns crop up over and over. Try Red Chestnut for fears about a baby's health or your relationship. Walnut might help you accept change and settle into your new state. Rock Water suits perfectionists who find it difficult to let go and enjoy simple pleasures. Put 2 drops of one or more remedies in a glass of water and sip throughout the day as needed.

Letting go

Pregnancy changes come easier if you let go a little: your body will do what it needs however hard you fight it – grow larger, get tired, not carry you far. Trying to lead your regular life can just leave you angry, frustrated and exhausted.

Don't try to do everything Hire a cleaner or decorator; tell the family you're not joining them for the holidays; turn down dinner parties, resign from committees.

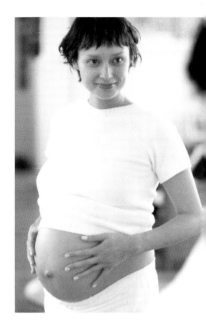

Lower your sights

Stop trying to be perfect at home and work, and don't try to do everything you did before pregnancy. In the last few weeks, plan on achieving less than one thing a day. It might only be sorting baby clothes or writing a birth plan.

Don't worry; be happy

Pregnancy makes you special. Some Muslims believe that when you are pregnant God "writes" against your name 1,000 good deeds and erases 1,000 bad deeds everyday.

Positive enjoyment

Sing

Especially good during pregnancy, singing strengthens the lungs, promotes deep breathing and good posture, focuses creativity and restores harmony with its own harmonies. Singing with a choir can be very calming: babies seem to kick or quieten with the vibrations of voices in unison. Sing lullabies to your baby from week 20. He can hear them now and they will calm him after the birth. Research shows babies quieten to the theme tune of a mother's favourite soap opera, associating the music with relaxation. Singing stimulates developing brain cells, too.

Garden

Plunging your hands into the earth and watching the seasons come and go is deeply reassuring as well as good exercise. (Wear gardening gloves to avoid coming in contact with any environmental toxins that can harm unborn babies.)

Paint, sew or knit

Absorption in a creative activity blocks other thoughts, and the more absorbed you become in the task, the more meditatively soothing the experience.

Read books, watch films

Escape your self-absorbed life for a hour or two while you can: cinemas and babies don't mix.

Pregnant not fat

To come to terms with the inevitable changes pregnancy brings, you need to adapt your attitude and that of those around you, because during pregnancy big is beautiful. In the UK, you'll not be routinely weighed at antenatal appointments, so avoid stepping on the bathroom scales, too. Free yourself from the guilt that usually accompanies weight gain, and if you're eating a well-balanced diet, enjoy the occasional cream cake or chocolate treat. See your new layer of padding, from puffy cheeks to swollen ankles, as vital nourishment and protection for your baby, imagining it becoming milk when you breastfeed. Discover the power of affirmations. Just saying out loud, "I love my bump" or "Big is beautiful" can have profound effects. Repeat it to yourself and others and soon you'll find you believe it. For the first time since adolescence, feel the freedom that comes with escaping the tyranny of the waistband. Flaunt your new cleavage and enjoy the woman-liness of your ample behind.

Dressing up

Rather than bemoaning the fact that nothing fits, see pregnancy as a shopping opportunity. You need pregnancy knickers and bras, hosiery and swimwear. Properly fitting foundation garments transform the way you feel about yourself by bringing comfort and shape; the self-confidence this instils is very empowering. Then comes outerwear: there is every reason to buy skirts and trousers with comfortable waistbands, dresses that won't rise up at the front and tops that don't strain over your breasts. Empire line and bias-cut are very flattering in pregnancy, and bodyhugging garments incredibly sexy. You don't have to spend a fortune; there are lots of affordable catwalk-inspired pregnancy lines and vintage is always cool. Also, try the Internet –

Peace amid flux

Being pregnant can make you question who you are: your parentage, your childhood and how you got to this point. Here is a meditative technique to help you work through such stressful thoughts.

1 Sit in a comfortable upright position, hands resting on your thighs. Close your eyes and take a few moments to calm and focus your mind by watching the waves of breath moving in and out.
2 When you feel tranquil, start to think about your body. Contemplate all the changes of pregnancy, trying to see the positive side of each one – love your new rolls of flesh for their ability to sustain your pregnancy and nourish your baby, for instance.
3 Ponder all the changes your body has undergone. Think of yourself inside your own mother's womb. Imagine your tiny fingers and toes when you were a newborn baby; visualize your chubby arms as a two-year-old; consider the changes of adolescence; imagine what you'll look like when your children have left home. Understand that the body is constantly in flux, that it does not define who you are.
4 Start to watch your mind. See it as a blank screen, then, without engaging with them, watch your thoughts projected on it. See how you remain at one remove from your thoughts. They are not you.
5 Next, notice sensations: pins and needles in your legs perhaps, a stuffy nose, sounds beyond the room. See how sensations change as time passes and understand that stimulation of the sense receptors is separate from you.
6 Appreciate the freedom of not having to be your body, thoughts or emotions. Appreciate yourself, unchanging, at the core of all this transformation.

eBay, for example, always has some interesting items. Friends with new babies will be only too glad to give away the clothes they lived in for months.

Enjoying your body

If you feel good about your body, you're more likely to feel turned on to the wonderful opportunities for passion that pregnancy can bring. Freed from worry about contraception or conception, many women find this a liberating time sexually, when it's possible to indulge your expansive body and newly awakened senses, experimenting with new sexual positions that make the most of your bump, butt and breasts.

Stop listening to others

When you're pregnant, you become public property. The world feels it has the right to stroke your belly, foretell the sex of your child, relate horror stories about birth and scowl at you for ordering a take-away latte, let alone sipping a glass of wine. To avoid toxic overload, smile sweetly and change the subject, or just walk away like you never heard. Mix more with people you trust and who respect you.

Be cosseted

It's not natural to go through pregnancy alone. In India, Africa and the Far East, mothers-to-be are cared for by female relatives who take over onerous household tasks and offer massage, nutritious food and reassuring companionship and advice. Pregnant women are urged to take it easy and do only pleasant things, the belief being that this influences the nature of the unborn child. In the affluent West, we have lost this nurturing streak, and pregnant women are expected to carry on working and socializing as if nothing's changed. Even when you can't stop, it's important to take time each day to surround yourself with pleasant things. Treats seem more vital during the last weeks of pregnancy.

Pure essentials for the birth

Keep these next to your bed in a bag in the weeks leading up to your delivery date.

Face spritzer
Fill an atomizer bottle with water and chill (particularly good when you're in a hot birthing pool for hours), or buy specially blended products like Bellamama's Uplifting Face and Body Spritzer

Lip balm
When you breathe through your mouth for hours (days) on end, lips get sore and cracked. A salve blended from natural waxes, like jojoba, shea butter and beeswax, can save the day. Weleda's is scented with vanilla and rose. Spiezia's Organic's range is 100 percent organic.

Woollen socks and slippers
Keep feet warm while you pace the corridor; during labour, extremities can get cold (you don't need more discomfort at this point). Schmidt's slippers are felted in pure water without chemicals and have natural rubber soles.

Washable nursing pads/nipple cream
Organic cotton is the new favourite, though naturally microbial hemp might suit better, since it's more absorbent and breathable. Scandinavian mums swear by Lana's Danish Pads made from untreated merino wool (*www.danishwool.com*). The natural lanolin has antibacterial

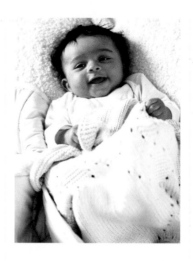

qualities. Schmidt recommends 50 percent untreated silk/50 percent merino wool for the fabrics' healing properties. For a nipple cream, choose one yummy enough to eat, like Earth Mama Angel Baby's Natural Nipple Butter.

Organic blankets and hooded towels
Wrap your tiny mite in Under the Nile's blanket or hooded bath towel, Schmidt's extra-thick, unbleached, undyed, untreated brushed cotton or a vintage Shetland knitted shawl (there were no pesticides in the 19th century!).

Gentle soap
For showering after birth, choose bars delicate enough for mother and baby, such as Jurlique's Body Bars and Weleda's Calendula Baby Soap.

Perineum repair kit
Witch hazel or arnica-based potions are antidotes for the swelling and

soreness following episiotomies, tears and general bruising. Try misting with the sweet-scented New Mama Bottom Spray or a smear of cooling Bottom Balm, both from Earth Mama Angel Baby.

Organic sanitary towels
Natracare's extra long and absorbent sanitary pads are non-chlorine-bleached cotton. They do not contain irritant absorbents, fragrance or optical whiteners and are less likely to irritate sore skin.

Organic nursing gown
Under the Nile's organic Egyptian cotton ensures your newborn's skin isn't irritated unnecessarily as he lies in your arms.

Non-tox baby lotion and nappy change cream
Try Weleda's, made from sesame oil, or Burt's Bees Baby Bees': as effective for your skin as baby's. Take along an organic nappy salve (Spiezia's is the best I've found, Baby Bee Skin Crème with borax fine, too) to prevent unenlightened neonatal nurses plastering inch-thick layers of petrochemicals over your precious baby's brand-new bottom.

Organic baby clothes and cot sheets
Prewash in eco washing liquid – as newborn skin doesn't thicken until 3-5 days after birth, it's more permeable and susceptible to absorbing toxins from dyes and disinfectants.

Index

Acknowledgments

The author would like to thank: contributing homeopath Julia Linfoot (*juliahomeopath@hotmail.com*); herbalist Peter Jackson-Main (*www.thenaturalcentre.com*) and labour aromatherapist Jane Tilton, Peckham Pulse Health Zone, London SE15 4QF).

Thanks to all the natural product companies who supplied information and samples (most of whom can arrange international delivery, by the way, and their stuff is fab), especially The Organic Pharmacy, Living Nature, REN, Jurlique, Weleda, Bella Mama, Earth Mama Angel Baby, Burt's Bees, Natalia, Spiezia Organics, Green People, Schmidt Natural Clothing, Natural Collection, Ecover, Seventh Generation, Howies, Circaroma, Avea, Elemis, Dr. Hauschka, Gossypium.

Special thanks to all those who shared knowledge and time, including Margo Marrone, Glenn Kositzki-Metzner, Gregor Barnum, Tim Madeley and Barb at Earth Mama Angel Baby. Thanks also to Mary, Georgia, Salima and Stacey for testing products.

Carroll & Brown would like to thank:
Computer Management: Paul Stradling
Picture Researcher: Sandra Schneider

Picture Credits
page 22 www.naturalcollection.com
page 29 www.circaroma.com
page 34 (top) courtesy of Dr. Hauschka;
(bottom) www.elemis.com
page 44 www.avea.co.uk
page 56 Norbert Schaefer/Corbis
page 76 Janine Hosegood/Courtesy of
Dr. Hauschka
page 94 www.greenfibres.com